Biocompatibility of Dental Biomaterials

Related titles

Cellular Response to Biomaterials,
(ISBN: 978-1-84569-358-9)

Materials Science for Dentistry,
(ISBN: 978-1-84569-529-3)

Non-Metallic Biomaterials for Tooth Repair and Replacement
(ISBN: 978-0-85709-244-1)

Woodhead Publishing Series in Biomaterials

Biocompatibility of Dental Biomaterials

Edited by

Richard Shelton

ELSEVIER

AMSTERDAM • BOSTON • HEIDELBERG • LONDON
NEW YORK • OXFORD • PARIS • SAN DIEGO
SAN FRANCISCO • SINGAPORE • SYDNEY • TOKYO
Woodhead Publishing is an imprint of Elsevier

WP WOODHEAD PUBLISHING

Woodhead Publishing is an imprint of Elsevier
The Officers' Mess Business Centre, Royston Road, Duxford, CB22 4QH, United Kingdom
50 Hampshire Street, 5th Floor, Cambridge, MA 02139, United States
The Boulevard, Langford Lane, Kidlington, OX5 1GB, United Kingdom

British Library Cataloguing-in-Publication Data
A catalogue record for this book is available from the British Library

Library of Congress Cataloging-in-Publication Data
A catalog record for this book is available from the Library of Congress

ISBN: 978-0-08-100884-3 (print)
ISBN: 978-0-08-100943-7 (online)

For information on all Woodhead Publishing visit our website at https://www.elsevier.com

Publisher: Matthew Deans
Acquisition Editor: Laura Overend
Editorial Project Manager: Lucy Beg
Production Project Manager: Poulouse Joseph
Designer: Maria Inês Cruz

Typeset by MPS Limited, Chennai, India

Contents

List of Figures

List of Tables

List of Contributors

A. Ballo University of British Columbia, Vancouver, BC, Canada

G. Ben-Gal The Hebrew University-Hadassah School of Dental Medicine, Jerusalem, Israel

N. Beyth The Hebrew University-Hadassah School of Dental Medicine, Jerusalem, Israel

W. Brantley The Ohio State University, Columbus, OH, United States

G. Gómez-Moreno University of Granada, Granada, Spain

Y. Houri-Haddad The Hebrew University-Hadassah School of Dental Medicine, Jerusalem, Israel

G. Iezzi University "G. d'Annunzio", Chieti, Italy

K. Moharamzadeh University of Sheffield, Sheffield, United Kingdom

P. Murray Nova Southeastern University College of Dental Medicine, Fort Lauderdale, FL, United States

T. Närhi University of Turku, Turku, Finland; Turku University Central Hospital, Turku, Finland

C.H. Pameijer Emeritus Professor, University of Connecticut, Farmington, CT, United States

V. Perrotti University "G. d'Annunzio", Chieti, Italy

A. Piattelli University "G. d'Annunzio", Chieti, Italy

Y. Pietrokovski The Hebrew University-Hadassah School of Dental Medicine, Jerusalem, Israel

A. Quaranta Oral Health Centre of Western Australia, Nedlands, WA, Australia

K.R. St. John University of Mississippi Medical Center, Jackson, MS, United States

Y. Uçar Cukurova University, Balcali, Adana, Turkey

A. Zabrovsky The Hebrew University-Hadassah School of Dental Medicine, Jerusalem, Israel

Biocompatibility of dental biomaterials

1

V. Perrotti[1], *A. Piattelli*[1], *A. Quaranta*[2], *G. Gómez-Moreno*[3] *and G. Iezzi*[1]
[1]University "G. d'Annunzio", Chieti, Italy; [2]Oral Health Centre of Western Australia, Nedlands, WA, Australia; [3]University of Granada, Granada, Spain

Chapter Outline

1.1 Introduction

Biocompatibility is the ability of a material to elicit an appropriate biological response to a given application in the body. Biocompatibility is not a property of just the material, but rather a property of how the material reacts with its environment. Indeed, Williams in 2008 defined biocompatibility as: "the ability of a biomaterial to perform its desired function with respect to a medical therapy, without eliciting any undesirable local or systemic effects in the recipient or beneficiary of that therapy, but generating the most appropriate beneficial cellular or tissue response to that specific situation, and optimizing the clinically relevant performance of that therapy."

The most recent thinking regarding biocompatibility is that it is possible to customize interactions at the material–tissue interface. Therefore, several factors must be considered when trying to measure the biological response. The most important factors include:

- *Location of the material*: this is important to its overall biological response. In general, materials that communicate through the epitheliuim or lie completely beneath it will need closer scrutiny when assessing the biological response than materials that do not penetrate the epithelium. Similarly, materials that penetrate tooth enamel will need more scrutiny than materials than do not. The surroundings of a material can be soft tissue or hard tissue; the material can be exposed directly to the blood, tissue fluids, or saliva, or through a barrier; the material can be placed externally or internally to the oral epithelium.
- *Duration of material in the body*: the duration of the presence of a material in the body is important to the biological response because many interactive effects between the body and material take time to develop. In general, the most stringent tests to measure biocompatibility

Biocompatibility of Dental Biomaterials. DOI: http://dx.doi.org/10.1016/B978-0-08-100884-3.00001-1

are required for materials that are present for the longest durations. Long durations give sufficient time for the material to affect the body and for the body to affect the material in many complex ways. What happens when grafted biomaterials and/or dental implants remain in the body for a long time period? Many biomaterials have been proposed in bone regeneration procedures in the oral cavity and in the jaws (Iezzi et al., 2012). Some biomaterials are synthetic, while others have a biologic origin. Some of them, e.g., calcium sulfate, beta-tricalcium phosphate, or polylactic/polyglycolic acid, are resorbed in humans within a few months (3–6 months); however, some biomaterials, e.g. hydroxyapatite, or anorganic bovine bone (ABB), can remain in the grafted healed site for long periods (years or even decades). One of the questions that could be asked concerns a possible negative, untoward effect of the persistence of these biomaterials in the grafted sites on the bone regeneration processes. The long-term fate of some biomaterials is still unknown and the reports present in the literature are not conclusive regarding whether these biomaterials are resorbed over time or not. Different reports can be found regarding the resorption behavior of different biomaterials, e.g. of ABB, one of the most commonly used biomaterials (Perrotti et al., 2009a,b). A group of researchers found that ABB resorbs over time (Galindo-Moreno et al., 2013). The resorption rate of ABB in vivo has been reported to be 2–3 years, and a decrease of about 10% per year has been reported. Other researchers have found that the potential metabolization of ABB by osteoclasts can be confirmed by the progressive increase in relative bone volume. Moreover, it has been reported that the density of ABB decreases by a little more than 10% between 6 and 12 months, suggesting a slow, but active resorption. ABB has been found to become integrated, and subsequently replaced, by newly formed bone. Conversely, other researchers found no signs of ABB resorption even after many years. Our group reported the persistence of biomaterials (hydroxyapatite, ABB) in the grafted sites after many years (7, 9, 14, or even after 2 decades) (Degidi et al., 2013; Iezzi et al., 2007). No untoward effects on bone regeneration processes were ever observed. An ideal material should provide a framework for continuous bone resorption and bone deposition. There is a hypothesis that the presence of graft particles at about 25–30% of the treated site volume may interfere with normal healing, while revascularization and nourishment are deprived, and this could cause problems in the osseointegration of dental implants inserted in these sites. Our histological results of implants inserted in sites regenerated, e.g., with ABB and retrieved after many years (4, 5, 8 years), disprove this notion, because we found in all these case reports a high percentage of bone–implant contact percentage (between 50 and 80%) with mineralized tissue at the interface of these implants even after long loading periods. ABB resorption does not seem to be absolutely necessary to provide predictable osseointegration. The almost complete incorporation of the ABB particles in bone could, however, produce a composite of structural bone–grafted particles creating a dense, hard tissue network around an implant. This network could provide a strong support to loaded dental implants, which is comparable to or even exceeds the support provided by native bone. Moreover, ABB could offer a long-term stress shield against pressure from the overlying gingival or sinus mucosa and the resistance of ABB to resorption and degradation may be advantageous for maintaining the initial dimensions of the augmented area with time. Furthermore, in some clinical situations a low substitution rate may be beneficial, because the physical support from the graft material helps to maintain the augmented volume and to prevent soft tissue collapse.

Histological analysis of human-retrieved implants is certainly a very useful tool to evaluate the bone implant contact percentage (BIC%), the implant biocompatibility and osteoconductivity after a long implantation time (Iezzi et al., 2016). Moreover, additional information can be gained on the biological reaction of the peri-implant tissues and on the bone turnover (modeling/remodeling) over a long-term period. It is believed that a very important factor for the long-term success of an implant, could be an adequate continuous remodeling of the peri-implant mineralized tissues. Human-retrieved implants, after functional periods of several years, have shown changes in the peri-implant bone microstructure, due to correlations between compressive stresses and collagen fiber orientation. Continuous bone remodeling was frequently observed in loaded implants even after almost three decades. The remodeling cycles help to obtain a very high level of organization with very good mechanical properties of the peri-implant bone. Even after many years or a few decades of functional loading, the implants appeared to be well integrated and demonstrated a very high and more than adequate BIC%, with no signs of the presence of connective fibrous tissue at the interface or epithelial downgrowth. Haversian systems were observed frequently close to the implant bone interface, showing that the bone was undergoing remodeling. In conclusion, data from human specimens showed that these implants had the potential to maintain osseointegration under long-term function, with continuous and ongoing peri-implant bone remodeling.

- *Stresses placed on the material*: these are important to the biological response. Stresses may be physical, chemical, or thermal in nature. Short-term, long-term, and fatigue stresses all need to be considered when assessing the effects of stress on the biological performance of materials.

1.2 Measuring the biocompatibility of dental biomaterials

Measuring the biocompatibility of a material is not simple. The methods of measurement are evolving rapidly as more becomes known about the interactions between dental materials and oral tissues and as technologies for testing improve. The evaluation of the biocompatibility of dental materials is a complex and comprehensive area because a great variety of different types of unwanted tissue reactions may occur. Practitioners should understand that there are no inert materials. When material is placed into living tissue, interactions with the complex biologic systems around it occur, and those interactions result in some sort of biologic response.

Historically, new materials were simply tried in humans to see whether they demonstrated biocompatibility. However, this practice has not been acceptable for many years, and current materials must be extensively screened for biocompatibility before they are ever used in humans. Nowadays, the common approach and principle, when testing the biological behavior of materials, is to start with simple in vitro tests mostly based on cell cultures, as is generally done in toxicology. If these experiences and investigations of a material's efficiency deliver promising findings, then more comprehensive studies on experimental animals and usage tests (in vivo evaluation) will be performed. Clinical studies are the final step of this evaluation process (Schmalz and Arenholt-Bindslev, 2008). In a recent review by Hulsart-Billström et al., a surprisingly poor correlation between in vitro and in vivo testing of biomaterials for bone regeneration was found as the result of a multicentre analysis. The outcomes of the in vitro and in vivo experiments were scored according to commonly recognized measures of success relevant to each experiment. The correlation of in vitro with in vivo scores for each assay alone and in combination was assessed and no significant correlation was found between in vitro and in vivo outcomes. The mean in vitro scores revealed a trend of covariance to in vivo scores of 58%. The inadequacies of the current in vitro assessments indicate the clear need for further development of novel approaches to relevant in vitro biomaterial testing and validated preclinical pipelines. In conclusion, there is a considerable need for proven in vitro assays that are able to reduce the burden on animal testing, by allowing assessment of biomaterial utility predictive of the results currently obtained through in vivo studies (Hulsart-Billström

Table 1.1 Summary of different available tests to measure the biocompatibility of a material

	Definition	Types	Advantages	Disadvantages
In vitro tests	In vitro test are performed with microorganisms, cells or biological molecules outside a living organism (test tube, cell culture dish, etc.)	*Direct tests*: material contacts the cell system without barrier • Cytotoxicity test • Membrane permeability test • Test for cell metabolism or cell function • MTT test • Mutagenesis assays *Indirect tests*: there is a barrier of some sort between the material and the cell system • Agar overlay method • Millipore filter assay • Dentin barrier tests	**1.** Quick to perform **2.** Least expensive **3.** Can be standardized **4.** Large scale screening **5.** Good experimental control **6.** Excellence for mechanism of interaction	**1.** Relevance to the final in vivo use is questionable **2.** Lack if inflammatory and other tissue protection mechanisms in the in vitro environment **3.** Cannot predict the overall biocompatibility of a material
In vivo tests	In vivo tests are those in which the effects of various biological entities are assessed on whole, living organisms, usually animals	• Mucous membrane irritation test • Skin sensitization test • Implantation tests • Maximization test	**1.** More relevant than in vitro tests, difficult to interpret and control	**1.** Expensive **2.** Time consuming, **3.** Involves significant ethical concern
Usage tests	Usage tests are performed in human study participants and require that the material be placed in a situation identical to its intended clinical use	• Dental pulp irritation tests • Periapical tissue damage and endodontic usage test • Dental implants in bone • Mucosa and gingival usage tests • Allergic responses to dental materials	**1.** Highly predictable for biocompatibility **2.** Fidelity to mimic the clinical use, including time, location, environment, and placement technique	**1.** Very expensive **2.** Very time consuming **3.** Major legal/ethical issues **4.** Can be difficult to control **5.** Difficult to interpret and quantify

et al., 2016). Currently, biocompatibility is measured by: (1) in vitro tests; (2) animal tests; (3) usage tests (see Table 1.1). Any single test method is applicable only for investigating one type of unwanted reaction out of a great variety of possible reactions. For example, cell culture tests will detect only the influence of a material on isolated cells. These findings cannot be transferred to patients without limitations. Indeed, an alloy that does not cause a reaction in cell culture may result in problems in patients because the patients may have a lower pH value in the oral cavity; this lower pH may result in a more pronounced corrosion of the alloy in vivo compared to the neutral conditions in cell culture.

Clinical investigations and observations as well as animal studies, mainly on larger animals such as primates or dogs, are used to investigate the potential harmfulness of a biomaterial for the patient or dental personnel. The animal models are adequate for the best possible simulations of a material's application in patients (usage tests) (Figs. 1.1–1.4).

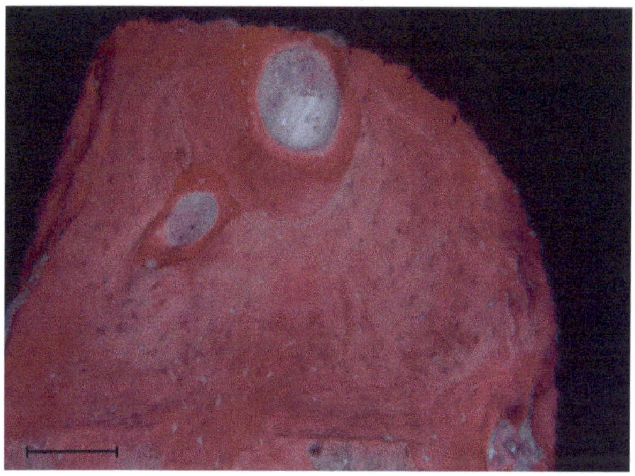

Figure 1.1 There are no gaps at the interface between the bone and the implant surface. Staining: toluidine blue and acid fuchsin (scale bar 100 μm).

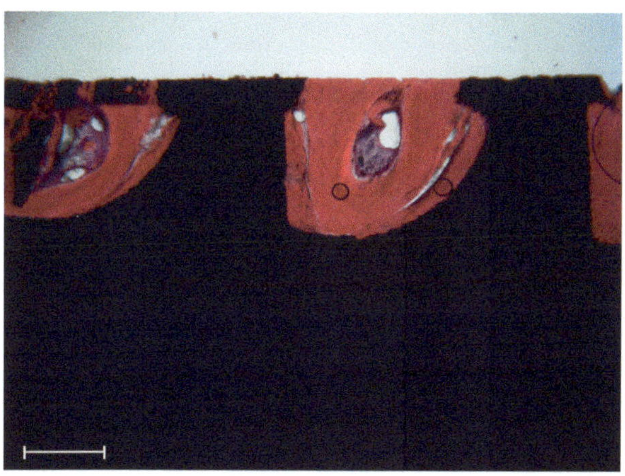

Figure 1.2 The concavities of the implant threads are completely filled by bone after more than 5 years of loading. Staining: toluidine blue and acid fuchsin (scale bar 400 μm).

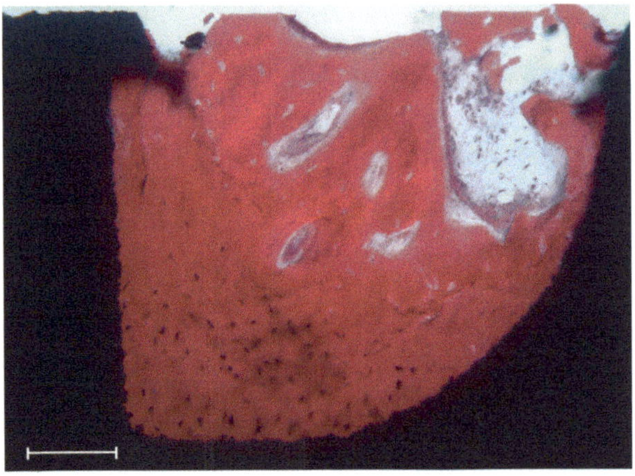

Figure 1.3 Osteocyte lacunae filled by osteocytes in the vicinity of the implant surface. Staining: toluidine blue and acid fuchsin (scale bar 100 μm).

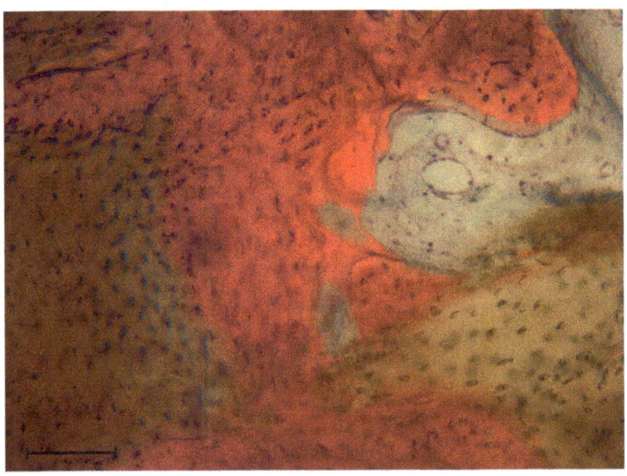

Figure 1.4 After 3 years, the anorganic bovine bone particles appear to have been incorporated into the bone, producing a sort of composite bone–graft structure. Staining: toluidine blue and acid fuchsin (scale bar 100 μm).

References

Degidi, M., Perrotti, V., Piattelli, A., Iezzi, G., 2013. Eight-year results of site retention of anorganic bovine bone and anorganic bovine matrix. J. Oral Implantol. 39 (6), 727–732.

Galindo-Moreno, P., Hernández-Cortés, P., Mesa, F., Carranza, N., Juodzbalys, G., Aguilar, M., et al., 2013. Slow resorption of anorganic bovine bone by osteoclasts in maxillary sinus augmentation. Clin. Implant Dent. Relat. Res. 15 (6), 858–866.

Hulsart-Billström, G., Dawson, J.I., Hofmann, S., Müller, R., Stoddart, M.J., Alini, M., et al., 2016. A surprisingly poor correlation between in vitro and in vivo testing of biomaterials for bone regeneration: results of a multicentre analysis. Eur. Cell. Mater. 31, 312–322. 24.

Iezzi, G., Degidi, M., Scarano, A., Petrone, G., Piattelli, A., 2007. Anorganic bone matrix retrieved 14 years after a sinus augmentation procedure: a histologic and histomorphometric evaluation. J. Periodontol. 78 (10), 2057–2061.

Iezzi, G., Degidi, M., Piattelli, A., Mangano, C., Scarano, A., Shibli, J.A., et al., 2012. Comparative histological results of different biomaterials used in sinus augmentation procedures: a human study at 6 months. Clin. Oral Implants Res. 23 (12), 1369–1376.

Iezzi, G., Piattelli, A., Mangano, C., Degidi, M., Testori, T., Vantaggiato, G., et al., 2016. Periimplant Bone Response in Human-Retrieved, Clinically Stable, Successful, and Functioning Dental Implants After a Long-Term Loading Period: A Report of 17 Cases From 4 to 20 Years. Implant Dent. 25 (3), 380–386.

Perrotti, V., Nicholls, B.M., Horton, M.A., Piattelli, A., 2009a. Human osteoclast formation and activity on a xenogenous bone mineral. J. Biomed. Mater Res. A 90 (1), 238–246.

Perrotti, V., Nicholls, B.M., Piattelli, A., 2009b. Human osteoclast formation and activity on an equine spongy bone substitute. Clin. Oral Implants Res. 20 (1), 17–23. Available from http://dx.doi.org/10.1111/j.1600-0501.2008.01608.x.

Schmalz, G., Arenholt-Bindslev, D., 2008. Determination of biocompatibility. In: Schmalz, G. (Ed.), Biocompatibility of Dental Materials. Springer Berlin Heidelberg, Germany, pp. 13–43.

Williams, D.F., 2008. On the mechanisms of biocompatibility. Biomaterials 29 (20), 2941–2953.

Mechanical biocompatibility of dental materials

2

K.R. St. John
University of Mississippi Medical Center, Jackson, MS, United States

Abstract

Materials used in dental restoration, implant dentistry, maxillofacial trauma and reconstruction, and other surgeries to correct or repair the mandible and maxilla do not have the same mechanical properties as the natural tissues. An area of concern in terms of the long-term success of procedures conducted by dentists and oral surgeons is the impact of differences in the mechanical properties of natural tissues and those of materials used for reconstruction on the response of tissues as healing occurs. The factors which may impact success and possible partial solutions are discussed.

Chapter Outline

Biocompatibility of Dental Biomaterials. DOI: http://dx.doi.org/10.1016/B978-0-08-100884-3.00002-3

2.1 Introduction

The term "biocompatibility" is frequently construed in the narrow sense of the nature of the biological response to the materials, either alloplastic or biologically derived. These materials may be used in construction of an oral or dental device, fixed or removable prosthodontics appliances, or in direct restoration of tooth structure. Additionally, materials may be used in auxiliary applications, such as for impressions, or to maintain exposure or dryness of the operative site. Mechanical compatibility is a different way of looking at the interactions between materials and devices used in dental practice and oral surgery, encompassing the consideration of the mechanical properties of the materials and devices and the ways in which tissues respond to these mechanical properties. It also involves the matching of the properties of materials with the tissues in which they will be placed to maintain, as closely as possible, normal function of the combined natural and restorative system while maximizing the longevity of the repair or replacement. This concept often results in quasi-compatibility because the requirements of the application necessitate using a material which may exhibit some desirable properties while sacrificing others to attain the overall best functional outcome.

Included in Table 2.1 are the properties of a subset of materials that may be encountered in restorative dentistry or oral surgery, either as the naturally present tissue or as materials used to restore form, function, and esthetics.

2.1.1 Restorative materials

Materials used in the restoration of form and function to carious or damaged tooth structure range from reinforced polymeric composite materials to formed-in-place metal alloys (amalgam), base metal and precious metal alloys, and ceramics. These may include cavity filling materials, crowns, bridges, dentures, and the masticatory and exposed portions of constructs supported by dental implants. For anterior restorations, esthetic considerations may overshadow or impact materials selection based upon mechanical properties, while there may be more flexibility in material selection in posterior restorations. These materials must maintain the sealing of the margins of the restorations, withstand the masticatory forces without fatigue or fracture, and lead to as little wear as possible, both of the restoration itself and of the opposing materials, either natural or synthetic, with which occlusion occurs. Maximal masticatory forces were reported in 1991 (Van Eijden, 1991) to be as high as approximately 725N. More recently, studies and finite element models have suggested that masticatory forces could be over 1200N (Koc et al., 2010; Demenko et al., 2011; Wroe et al., 2010).

2.1.2 Orthodontics

The correction of malpositioned teeth and malocclusion requires that force be placed on the teeth over time, allowing them to be moved into the appropriate positions. The materials used in orthodontic brackets and wires must withstand the forces placed upon them by the practitioner at the time of placement or adjustment, as well as

Table 2.1 Typical mechanical properties of dental and orofacial materials

Material	Elastic modulus (GPa)	Tensile strength (MPa)	Flexural strength (MPa)	Compressive strength (MPa)	Yield strength (MPa)	Hardness (GPa)
Bone	17	133		193	114	0.234–0.760
Enamel	84	10		262		3.0–3.6
Dentin	17	106		234		0.57–0.66
Amalgam	21	27–55		189		1.08–1.87
Composite resin materials	17–21	25–90		225		
Dental porcelain	40–70	50–100	60–80	150–175		4.5
Leucite-based ceramics			120			
Lithium disilicate ceramics	110		250–300			
Zirconia (3Y-TZP)	210		800–1300			13–13.5
Zirconia			630			
Alumina	350	120	600–700			
Commercially pure titanium	104	550			485	
Ti-6Al-4V	105	900			835	
Gold alloys	90–95	490			400	
Cobalt–chromium dental alloys	184	1700			1400	3.83
Nickel–chromium dental alloys	154–210	540–1360			260–840	
Stainless steel	179	2100			1600	
Nickel–titanium	41	1500			430	
PEEK (poly(ether ether ketone))	4	93				

Source: Adapted from Anusavice, K.J., 2003. Mechanical properties of dental materials. In: Anusavice, K.J. (Ed.), Phillips' Science of Dental Materials. Eleventh ed. St. Louis, MO: Saunders (Anusavice, 2003); Braga, R.R., Pfeifer, C.S., Sakaguchi, R.L., 2012. Testing of dental materials and biomechanics. In: Sakaguchi, R.L., Powers, J.M. (Eds.), Craig's Restorative Dental Materials. Thirteenth ed. Philadelphia, PA: Mosby (Braga et al., 2012); Brantley, W.A., 2003. Wrought alloys. In: Anusavice, K.J. (Ed.), Phillips' Science of Dental Materials. Eleventh ed. St. Louis, MO: Saunders (Brantley, 2003); Anusavice, K.J., Brantley, W.A., 2003. Physical properties of dental materials. In: Anusavice, K.J. (Ed.), Phillips' Science of Dental Materials. Eleventh ed. St. Louis, MO: Saunders (Anusavice and Cascone, 2003); Denry, I.L., 2012. Restorative materials—ceramics. In: Sakaguchi, R.L., Powers, J.M. (Eds.), Craig's Restorative Dental Materials. Thirteenth ed. Philadelphia, PA: Mosby (Denry, 2012); Reilly, D.T., Burstein, A.H., 1975. The elastic and ultimate properties of compact bone tissue. J. Biomech. 8, 393–405 (Reilly and Burstein, 1975); Bayraktar, H.H., Morgan, E.F., Niebur, G.L., Morris, G.E., Wong, E.K., Keaveny, T.M., 2004. Comparison of the elastic and yield properties of human femoral trabecular and cortical bone tissue. J. Biomech. 37, 27–35. doi:10.1016/S0021-9290(03)00257-4 (Bayraktar et al., 2004); Zysset, P.K., Edward GUO, X., Edward Hoffler, C., Moore, K.E., Goldstein, S.A., 1999. Elastic modulus and hardness of cortical and trabecular bone lamellae measured by nanoindentation in the human femur. J. Biomechan. 32, 1005–1012, doi:10.1016/S0021-9290(99)00111-6 (Zysset et al., 1999); Hasheminezhad, A., Zebarjad, S.M., Sajjadi, S.A., Rahanjam, L., 2012. Effect of copper content on compressive strength and microstructure of dental amalgams. Engineering 4, 155–159, doi:10.4236/eng.2012.43020 (Hasheminezhad et al., 2012); Turp, V., Tuncelli, B., Sen, D., Goller, G., 2012. Evaluation of hardness and fracture toughness, coupled with microstructural analysis, of zirconia ceramics stored in environments with different pH values. Dental Mater. J. 31, 891–902 (Turp et al., 2012); Kurtz, S.M., Devine, J.N., 2007. PEEK biomaterials in trauma, orthopedic, and spinal implants. Biomaterials 28, 4845–4869. doi:10.1016/j.biomaterials.2007.07.013 (Kurtz and Devine, 2007); Niinomi, M., 1998. Mechanical properties of biomedical titanium alloys. Mater. Sci. Eng. A 243, 231–236, doi:10.1016/S0921-5093(97)00806-X (Niinomi, 1998).

the forces that will be transmitted to them due to relative elastic movement of the teeth during mastication. Compared to the forces of mastication, the forces applied materials in orthodontic treatment are low, typically 25 gf (0.25N) to 225 gf (2.2N) (Roscoe et al., 2015), but the small cross-sections of the appliances used require careful consideration of the stresses in the materials (Proffit et al., 2013a,b). The brackets must securely retain the orthodontic springs and wires but allow repeated removal and adjustment of tension wires during treatment. The adhesive used to secure the brackets must be able to transfer loads to the teeth but allow removal of the brackets at the conclusion of treatment.

2.1.3 Materials for oral surgery

Materials used in oral surgery fall into several usage classifications, although the materials used in these applications are relatively consistent. The usages are divided into dental implants, devices for maintaining proper orientation of bone fragments and the temporary carriage of load after a maxillary or mandibular fracture, and devices used to stabilize bone fragments when orthognathic surgery is performed to correct deficiencies and deformities.

2.1.3.1 Dental implants

Dental implants serve as the primary structure carrying masticatory loads from the tooth crown to the bone of the maxilla or mandible when a missing tooth is being replaced. In order to function successfully, they must mechanically support the crown structure while transferring the loads to the underlying bone structure. As will be discussed later under stress protection atrophy, overloading or underloading of bone can lead to changes in bone structure that can lead to loss of support and failure of the prosthodontic appliance. These devices are used both to support a single tooth replacement and as proximal and distal supports for multiunit prosthetic devices.

2.1.3.2 Fracture fixation

Repairing damage to the mandible or maxilla due to trauma requires the use of devices to hold the fragments in place while healing occurs. These devices are usually plates and/or screws manufactured from stainless steel or titanium and its alloys. Additionally, wires may be used in conjunction with orthodontic brackets or screws to maintain a stable fracture reduction until bridging of the defects by bone has occurred. Frequently these materials must have high strength, high elastic modulus, and fatigue resistance to resist muscle forces and to carry the load of mastication if the patient will be allowed solid foods during healing. As discussed above, the masticatory forces may be as high as 1200N. Once healing has occurred, the high modulus materials can become a disadvantage because bone requires loading to fully heal and maintain its mass. If too much load is being carried by the devices, stress shielding can occur, leading to long-term loss of strength of the healed bone or necessitating the removal of the material after healing, in a second surgery.

2.1.3.3 Orthognathic surgery

This category of devices is, in reality, a subset of fracture fixation and orthodontia when it comes to devices and mechanical needs and challenges. Orthognathic surgery is usually elective to repair facial deformities or to correct malocclusion more severe than can be treated by orthodontic tooth movement, such as increasing or reducing the dimensions of the mandible or maxilla. Plates, screws, orthodontic brackets, and wires are all used to stabilize the bone which has been surgically separated, until healing occurs. Forces of mastication (if allowed by the surgeon) and forces generated by orofacial muscles must be carried by the fixation devices until healing has occurred and, at that time, it would be beneficial if loads could then be transferred to the healed bone instead of continuing to be carried by the devices and wires.

2.2 Challenges of mechanical biocompatibility in the oral environment

The oral environment, as with many other clinical environments, presents challenges because design for mechanical compatibility may be limited by other factors. One such factor is the fact that oral and maxillofacial surgery applications present a requirement that the design accommodate the size restrictions inherent in the mouth. In many industrial or infrastructure applications of materials, a design may incorporate the use of more material, creating a larger or more massive structure and reducing the stresses carried by the material. This cannot be done in oral applications because devices and restorations must fit with prepared tooth structure, comfortably adjacent to other tissue structures, such as cheeks, the palate, the tongue, within the confines of the bone structure of the mandible or maxilla, or buried between bone and soft tissue structures.

As seen in Table 2.1, natural materials and synthetic materials used in the oral environment exhibit a broad range of properties. When more than one natural material is being replaced or is the repository for synthetic materials, the most compatible material for interaction with one tissue may demonstrate adverse interactions with another material, meaning that trade-offs may have to be made, compromising what might appear, at first inspection, to be the best material for use.

2.2.1 Elastic modulus

By reference to Table 2.1, it can be seen that the elastic modulus of the materials used in dental and orofacial surgery may be significantly different from the modulus of enamel, bone, or dentin. Since the elastic modulus is a measure of the amount of elastic deformation that occurs when a defined amount of load is applied to the material, a mismatch between materials moduli may cause a difference in deformation when subjected to the same load or may cause the material with the higher modulus to carry a majority of the load. Alternatively, in designs and situations in which both materials carry the same load, differences in deformation may lead to loss of contact, retention, or marginal seal with repeated loading. As will be discussed further in relation to stress protection atrophy, the modulus of a material used in dental surgery may impact on the long-term success of the procedure being performed. Possibly the most challenging task in the selection of synthetic materials for bone contact or stabilization applications is that the vast majority of materials having different properties that make them suitable for use have elastic moduli that are significantly above that of either cancellous or cortical bone. In Table 2.1, the only materials listed with an elastic modulus similar to bone are the composite resin materials. These are typically used as restorative materials and not bone implant materials, although other designs of composite materials, not listed, have been investigated for bone implant and bone stabilization applications outside of the oral applications.

2.2.2 Strength

Strength is possibly the material property that would most frequently come to mind when considering mechanical biocompatibility of a dental material. The materials used in all areas of dental and oral surgery must be capable of withstanding the forces experienced during clinical use without fracture or permanent deformation. While this may be an obvious requirement, meeting this requirement necessitates defining the loading that will be transferred to devices and restorations under not only normal usage, but also incorporates the careful definition of worst-case conditions to which a patient might subject the material under any foreseeable circumstance of usage or misuse. It may not be possible to address the loading requirements of extremely unlikely high-load situations while maintaining other design characteristics that are important under normal usage, but it is important to at least consider high load possibilities. There is, however, a need for a safety factor of over-design which will partially account for unexpected higher loading. Additionally, as will be discussed next, failure of materials can occur at loading levels below that of the strength determined by the single application of a load to the point of failure.

2.2.3 Fatigue resistance

In a majority of medical device mechanical failures in usage, fracture does not occur as a result of a single overloading of the material, but due to fatigue. The oral environment is one in which loads are applied repetitively and this can occur in a restorative or other dental material for periods as long as 50 or more years. A material that is repetitively subjected to loads that are only a fraction of the material strength will usually undergo formation of one or more microscopic cracks that can then progress through the material by a very small amount with each cycle of loading, with this crack propagation occurring over thousands or hundreds of thousands of loading cycles. As crack propagation occurs, the actual cross-section withstanding the load is reduced with each cycle until failure then occurs over very few cycles as the stress experienced by the remaining cross-section exceeds the strength of the material.

In addition to the repetitive loading of mastication, the clasps and other retention features of removable prosthodontic appliances undergo repeated elastic deformation upon placement and removal, as well as repetitive bending stresses depending upon design and other retention features of the appliance.

The fatigue limit (endurance limit) of a material is the level of stress that can be sustained without failure when loading is applied repeatedly. If such a limit exists, it is usually less than 50% of the strength of the material and below the yield strength. Many times, testing will show that there is not an upper limit of stress that can be called a fatigue limit but, rather, a stress which can be sustained for a specified period, such as ten million cycles.

Materials selected for use in restorative applications, temporary support applications, such as trauma, or implant applications must be compatible with the loading regime to which they will be subjected and materials which undergo failure in fatigue under normal usage conditions should be considered noncompatible with the application being considered, except for situations in which it is known that the material will be removed from service or load bearing before failure occurs.

2.2.4 Hardness and wear

The mechanical properties of restorative materials in the oral cavity may have a significant impact on the long-term maintenance of the integrity of opposing surfaces during mastication. In the natural dentition, enamel is moving against enamel and therefore the abrasive interaction is between two materials of the same hardness. Referring to Table 2.1, it can be clearly seen that the hardness of materials used to form the chewing surfaces of natural teeth and alloplastic restorative materials includes a range of values. The table shows that the hardness of enamel is approximately double that of amalgam but one-quarter that of zirconia, while the hardness of dental porcelain can be similar to that of enamel. Hardness is not a direct measure of wear resistance but can provide valuable information about the likelihood of two opposing surface being compatible in wear. Differences in wear properties between opposing occlusal surface can have a deleterious effect on the long-term success of restorative procedures (Delong, 2006). A series of articles in *Dental Materials* in 2006 addressed the state of knowledge at that time, methods of simulating and quantifying wear, and the relative importance of wear being considered in selection of restorative materials (Delong, 2006; Ferracane, 2006; Heintze, 2006; Lambrechts et al., 2006).

The question of whether wear of dental composites was still a clinical concern was addressed (Ferracane, 2006) with a view to determine the need for wear simulation devices. The conclusion was that wear of larger composite restorations was still a clinical concern, particularly with habits that can accelerate wear, such as bruxing and the clenching of teeth. As a result, there remains a need to characterize the wear of new composites before clinical use in the laboratory. Delong (2006) addressed identifying the wear parameters that have clinical relevance and compared the use of the parameters of wear volume, wear depth (loss of height), and wear area as methods to quantify wear. It was concluded that volume was the best parameter to measure, both because it is a function of depth and area and because it has been found to be linear with time (and presumably amount of wear). In discussing methods for determining the volume of losses due to wear, it was suggested that the best method would be one which can be applied both clinically and in laboratory simulation. It was also proposed that a method which scans a three-dimensional image of the tooth and compares before and after images by subtraction would be very useful, assuming a before-wear image was available, which may be addressed by record impressions that have been cast in stone.

Two papers addressed the simulation and validation of wear simulation systems (Heintze, 2006; Lambrechts et al., 2006). It was determined that in vivo wear is a complex problem and it may be difficult to duplicate all appropriate characteristics in a simulator, and Lambrechts provided an overview of all of the simulators available at the time, their characteristics, including load, motion, mode of action, and lubricant. After a discussion of the physiological parameters that impact clinical wear, it was concluded with a summary of the advantages and disadvantages of extrapolating in vitro results in the prediction of clinical wear, without advocating one model of simulator over another. Heintze (2006) reported on the conduct of a round-robin test using 10 different restorative materials in 5 different simulators and concluded that wear quantitation methods can be validated but it was difficult to validate simulation methods and machines because of the lack of control of certain parameters and the lack of studies correlating simulator wear with actual clinical performance of the tested materials. Despite possible areas of necessary improvement in simulations, these methods are being used to compare the wear of restorative materials (Elmaria et al., 2006; Ghazal et al., 2008; Hacker et al., 1996; Heintze et al., 2008; Kadokawa et al., 2006; Mehl et al., 2007; Ramp et al., 1997; Stober et al., 2006).

2.2.5 Coefficient of thermal expansion

While not exactly a mechanical consideration, differences in expansion due to cycles of hot beverages and frozen items can lead to failure to maintain a tight margin around restorations, potentially allowing bacterial ingress and the development of secondary caries. If there is a sufficient difference in thermal expansion coefficient and a restoration expands more than the surrounding tooth structure upon warming, enough mechanical force can be generated to cause fracture of the tooth structure or partial creep or extrusion of the restorative material from the prepared cavity in the tooth (Anusavice and Brantley, 2003). With repeated temperature cycling, fatigue of the restorative material or tooth structure may also occur.

2.2.6 Stress protection atrophy of hard tissue

It is well known that bone undergoes continuous biological breakdown and redeposition as a part of the normal maintenance processes. These processes can be disrupted by diseases such as osteoporosis, leading to changes in the bone mass and morphology. The bone turnover process can also result in changes in bone mass and morphology in response to stresses that are placed on the bone. This is utilized in the movement of teeth in orthodontia and can be seen in the increases in bone mass that can occur in athletes as a response to the stresses placed on the bone in training and competition.

Bone remodels in response to stress by either increasing bone mass when there is an increase in the stresses it is required to carry or decreasing in form or mass as there is a decrease in the stresses being carried. When a medical device or appliance takes over a majority of the load-bearing responsibility from bone, the bone may remodel and a reduction in form or mass may occur, which is sometimes called "stress protection atrophy." While this might be a desirable outcome if the intent is a permanent implant or permanent replacement of function of the bone, this can become a great disadvantage if the bone is going to be expected to take over the load bearing later, such as for a fracture fixation device or a dental implant. Devices may be designed to interact with the normal bone anatomy, such as in a dental implant, but loss of bone may threaten the long-term success of the surgical intervention. The material property that is most closely related to concern for stress protection effects is the elastic modulus. The modulus of implant materials can be an order of magnitude greater than the modulus of bone, meaning that, when bone and an implant are working in parallel in a load-bearing application, a majority of the load will be carried by the implant material (Tonino et al., 1976). Titanium and its alloys are frequently chosen for bone contact applications for their osseointegration properties but they are theorized to be of advantage because the elastic modulus is only 5–6-times that of bone (Niinomi, 2008), rather than more than 10-times that of bone.

Several journal articles have focused on the potential for problems related to stress protection in dental applications (Asaoka et al., 1985; Kennady et al., 1989a,,b; Lee et al., 2012; Wiskott and Belser, 1999; Chen, 2012). The conclusions of these papers were that the stress protection effect does occur in dental implant applications and that design features, such as the selection of porous surfaces over smooth surfaces, and the investigation of polymeric materials as substitutes for metals may reduce the potential for problems to occur.

2.2.7 Integration of materials into hard tissues

Osseointegration has already been mentioned, but several aspects of the integration of materials into bone can have an impact on the success of bone contact applications. Titanium and its alloys can facilitate the transfer of load to bone because of the relatively unique characteristic of titanium in that a fibrous tissue interface does not normally form in healing, but rather tight apposition of bone to the metal surface occurs. Provision of porous coatings on the materials can allow the bone to grow into pores and ensure the transfer of loads to the bone when loads are placed upon the small islands of bone that are present in the pores. In addition, implant materials may be coated with bioactive ceramics such as hydroxyapatite to facilitate attachment of bone to the surfaces, so long as the mechanical properties of the coatings are such that their integrity is maintained with time, without either separating from the underlying material or becoming remodeled by the same biological organisms that participate in the turnover of bone.

2.3 Solutions

2.3.1 Material selection

One of the more obvious, but not necessarily simple solutions to problems of mechanical compatibility of dental and oromaxillofacial materials would be the selection of a material that has more desirable mechanical properties. Among the solutions being considered and tested is the use of PEEK (poly (ether ether ketone)) in dental applications (Lee et al., 2012; Schwitalla and Muller, 2013). Researchers have found that glass-fiber-reinforced PEEK has an elastic modulus similar to that of bone (Lee et al., 2012) and that the compressive strength might be adequate for anterior dental implants. The compressive strength of carbon-fiber-reinforced PEEK was nearly double that for the glass-fiber-reinforced material. Neither material had the strength of titanium devices, which is the material that is currently most commonly used. Further research on tunable composites and composite materials for applications in dentistry and oral surgery may yield other candidate materials for usage.

Another possible solution for improving the mechanical compatibility of titanium and its alloys may be creating bulk porosity of the material (Niinomi, 2008). The bulk elastic modulus of porous titanium was shown to be directly related to its porosity, achieving a modulus similar to that of bone at about 35% porosity. The trade-off for this potential solution was that the tensile strength and yield strength were also reduced. Similar research was also conducted at another research center (Asaoka et al., 1985), in which it was determined that creating the porosity in titanium was a biomechanically superior solution to trying to use low-modulus materials, such as polymers.

2.3.2 Surface modifications

As discussed above, changes in the surface properties, such as coatings and porosity, may improve the mechanical compatibility of a material in application. In recent years, there has also been research conducted to investigate whether the creation of microscopic surface morphology at the scale of the size of cells will affect how the cells react to the surface and create extracellular matrix. In the case of devices in contact with bone, this may hold the potential to change the way fibrous tissue or bone is deposited during healing.

2.3.3 Designing for compatibility

Porous coatings were mentioned as facilitators of bone ingrowth and stress transfer to bone but they also can be a design feature to impact the stresses at the interface between an implant and bone (Chen, 2012). In this study, finite element analysis was used to model the effects of a porous coating on a solid titanium device to ease the stress transfer to the bone, using the porous coating as a lower modulus material between bone and the solid titanium.

Elastic modulus is a material property but the design of a device with variation in cross section can be used to affect the stiffness of the device, which is a property of the device, i.e., while related to the material properties, tunable to some extent by the design parameters used in creation of a final component. The limitations of the site of usage and overall anatomy may cause this to be of limited application because of the other design requirements inherent in its usage.

2.4 Future trends

The future may hold many exciting opportunities to achieve better compatibility through the use of tissue engineering and stem cell techniques which may result in the creation of dental materials that actually are composed of the same natural substances which were originally compromised by the condition requiring treatment.

The possibilities of improving mechanical compatibility of existing materials that have been utilized in dental and oral surgery applications may be limited. For synthetic materials, advances in materials processing may provide some opportunities for improved properties but the trade-off in improving one material property is likely to induce changes in other properties which may or may not be beneficial to the application.

References

Anusavice, K.J., 2003. Mechanical properties of dental materials. In: Anusavice, K.J. (Ed.), Phillips' Science of Dental Materials, 11th ed. Saunders, St. Louis, MO.

Anusavice, K.J., Brantley, W.A., 2003. Physical properties of dental materials. In: Anusavice, K.J. (Ed.), Phillips' Science of Dental Materials, 11th ed. Saunders, St. Louis, MO.

Anusavice, K.J., Cascone, P., 2003. Dental casting and soldering alloys. In: Anusavice, K.J. (Ed.), Phillips' Science of Dental Materials., 11th ed. Saunders, St. Louis, MO.

Asaoka, K., Kuwayama, N., Okuno, O., Miura, I., 1985. Mechanical properties and biomechanical compatibility of porous titanium for dental implants. J. Biomed. Mater. Res. 19, 699–713. http://dx.doi.org/10.1002/jbm.820190609.

Bayraktar, H.H., Morgan, E.F., Niebur, G.L., Morris, G.E., Wong, E.K., Keaveny, T.M., 2004. Comparison of the elastic and yield properties of human femoral trabecular and cortical bone tissue. J. Biomech. 37, 27–35. http://dx.doi.org/10.1016/S0021-9290(03)00257-4.

Braga, R.R., Pfeifer, C.S., Sakaguchi, R.L., 2012. Testing of dental materials and biomechanics. In: Sakaguchi, R.L., Powers, J.M. (Eds.), Craig's Restorative Dental Materials, 13th ed. Mosby, Philadelphia, PA.

Brantley, W.A., 2003. Wrought alloys. In: Anusavice, K.J. (Ed.), Phillips' Science of Dental Materials, 11th ed. Saunders, St. Louis, MO.

Chen, L., 2012. Finite element analysis of the stress on the implant-bone interface of dental implants with different structures. In: Ebrahimi, F. (Ed.), Finite Element Analysis—New Trends and Developments. InTech, Rijeka.

Delong, R., 2006. Intra-oral restorative materials wear: Rethinking the current approaches: how to measure wear. Dental Mater. 22, 702–711. http://dx.doi.org/10.1016/j.dental.2006.02.003.

Demenko, V., Linetskiy, I., Nesvit, K., Shevchenko, A., 2011. Ultimate masticatory force as a criterion in implant selection. J. Dental Res. 90, 1211–1215. http://dx.doi.org/10.1177/0022034511417442.

Denry, I.L., 2012. Restorative materials—ceramics. In: Sakaguchi, R.L., Powers, J.M. (Eds.), Craig's Restorative Dental Materials., 13th ed. Mosby, Philadelphia, PA.

Elmaria, A., Goldstein, G., Vijayaraghavan, T., Legeros, R.Z., Hittelman, E.L., 2006. An evaluation of wear when enamel is opposed by various ceramic materials and gold. J. Prosth. Dentist. 96, 345–353. http://dx.doi.org/10.1016/j.prosdent.2006.09.002.

Ferracane, J.L., 2006. Is the wear of dental composites still a clinical concern?: is there still a need for in vitro wear simulating devices? Dental Mater. 22, 689–692. http://dx.doi.org/10.1016/j.dental.2006.02.005.

Ghazal, M., Yang, B., Ludwig, K., Kern, M., 2008. Two-body wear of resin and ceramic denture teeth in comparison to human enamel. Dental Mater. 24, 502–507. http://dx.doi.org/10.1016/j.dental.2007.04.012.

Hacker, C.H., Wagner, W.C., Razzoog, M.E., 1996. An in vitro investigation of the wear of enamel on porcelain and gold in saliva. J. Prosth. Dentist. 75, 14–17. http://dx.doi.org/10.1016/S0022-3913(96)90412-6.

Hasheminezhad, A., Zebarjad, S.M., Sajjadi, S.A., Rahanjam, L., 2012. Effect of copper content on compressive strength and microstructure of dental amalgams. Engineering 4, 155–159. http://dx.doi.org/10.4236/eng.2012.43020.

Heintze, S.D., 2006. How to qualify and validate wear simulation devices and methods. Dental Mater. 22, 712–734. http://dx.doi.org/10.1016/j.dental.2006.02.002.

Heintze, S.D., Cavalleri, A., Forjanic, M., Zellweger, G., Rousson, V., 2008. Wear of ceramic and antagonist—a systematic evaluation of influencing factors in vitro. Dental Mater. 24, 433–449. http://dx.doi.org/10.1016/j.dental.2007.06.016.

Kadokawa, A., Suzuki, S., Tanaka, T., 2006. Wear evaluation of porcelain opposing gold, composite resin, and enamel. J. Prosth. Dentist. 96, 258–265. http://dx.doi.org/10.1016/j.prosdent.2006.08.016.

Kennady, M.C., Tucker, M.R., Lester, G.E., Buckley, M.J., 1989a. Histomorphometric evaluation of stress shielding in mandibular continuity defects treated with rigid fixation plates and bone grafts. Int. J. Oral Maxillofac. Surg. 18, 170–174. http://dx.doi.org/10.1016/S0901-5027(89)80120-1.

Kennady, M.C., Tucker, M.R., Lester, G.E., Buckley, M.J., 1989b. Stress shielding effect of rigid internal fixation plates on mandibular bone grafts. A photon absorption densitometry and quantitative computerized tomographic evaluation. Int. J. Oral Maxillofac. Surg. 18, 307–310. http://dx.doi.org/10.1016/S0901-5027(89)80101-8.

Koc, D., Dogan, A., Bek, B., 2010. Bite force and influential factors on bite force measurements: a literature review. Eur. J. Dentist. 4, 223–232.

Kurtz, S.M., Devine, J.N., 2007. PEEK biomaterials in trauma, orthopedic, and spinal implants. Biomaterials 28, 4845–4869. http://dx.doi.org/10.1016/j.biomaterials.2007.07.013.

Lambrechts, P., Debels, E., Van Landuyt, K., Peumans, M., Van Meerbeek, B., 2006. How to simulate wear?: overview of existing methods. Dental Mater. 22, 693–701. http://dx.doi.org/10.1016/j.dental.2006.02.004.

Lee, W.-T., Koak, J.-Y., Lim, Y.-J., Kim, S.-K., Kwon, H.-B., Kim, M.-J., 2012. Stress shielding and fatigue limits of poly-ether-ether-ketone dental implants. J. Biomed. Mater. Res. B 100B, 1044–1052. http://dx.doi.org/10.1002/jbm.b.32669.

Mehl, C., Scheibner, S., Ludwig, K., Kern, M., 2007. Wear of composite resin veneering materials and enamel in a chewing simulator. Dental Mater. 23, 1382–1389. http://dx.doi.org/10.1016/j.dental.2006.11.026.

Niinomi, M., 1998. Mechanical properties of biomedical titanium alloys. Mater. Sci. Eng. A 243, 231–236. http://dx.doi.org/10.1016/S0921-5093(97)00806-X.

Niinomi, M., 2008. Mechanical biocompatibilities of titanium alloys for biomedical applications. J. Mech. Behav. Biomed. Mater. 1, 30–42. http://dx.doi.org/10.1016/j.jmbbm.2007.07.001.
Proffit, W.R., Fields, H.W., Sarver, D.M., 2013a. Chapter 9: Mechanical Principles in Orthodontic Force Control. Contemporary Orthodontics. Mosby, Canada.
Proffit, W.R., Fields, H.W., Sarver, D.M., 2013b. Chapter 14: The First Stage of Comprehensive Treatment: Alignment and Leveling Contemporary Orthodontics. Mosby, Canada.
Ramp, M.H., Suzuki, S., Cox, C.F., Lacefield, W.R., Koth, D.L., 1997. Evaluation of wear: enamel opposing three ceramic materials and a gold alloy. J. Prosth. Dentist. 77, 523–530. http://dx.doi.org/10.1016/S0022-3913(97)70146-X.
Reilly, D.T., Burstein, A.H., 1975. The elastic and ultimate properties of compact bone tissue. J. Biomech. 8, 393–405.
Roscoe, M.G., Meira, J.B.C., Cattaneo, P.M., 2015. Association of orthodontic force system and root resorption: A systematic review. Am. J. Orthodon. Dentofac. Orthoped. 147, 610–626. http://dx.doi.org/10.1016/j.ajodo.2014.12.026.
Schwitalla, A., Muller, W.-D., 2013. PEEK dental implants: a review of the literature. J. Oral Implantol. 39, 743–749.
Stober, T., Lutz, T., Gilde, H., Rammelsberg, P., 2006. Wear of resin denture teeth by two-body contact. Dental Mater. 22, 243–249. http://dx.doi.org/10.1016/j.dental.2005.03.009.
Tonino, A., Davidson, C., Klopper, P., Linclau, L., 1976. Protection from stress in bone and its effects. Experiments with stainless steel and plastic plates in dogs. J. Bone Joint Surgery, British Volume 58-B, 107–113.
Turp, V., Tuncelli, B., Sen, D., Goller, G., 2012. Evaluation of hardness and fracture toughness, coupled with microstructural analysis, of zirconia ceramics stored in environments with different pH values. Dental Mater. J. 31, 891–902.
Van Eijden, T.M.G.J., 1991. Three-dimensional analyses of human bite-force magnitude and moment. Arch. Oral Biol. 36, 535–539. http://dx.doi.org/10.1016/0003-9969(91)90148-N.
Wiskott, H.W.A., Belser, U.C., 1999. Lack of integration of smooth titanium surfaces: a working hypothesis based on strains generated in the surrounding bone. Clin. Oral Implan. Res. 10, 429–444. http://dx.doi.org/10.1034/j.1600-0501.1999.100601.x.
Wroe, S., Ferrara, T.L., Mchenry, C.R., Curnoe, D., Chamoli, U., 2010. The craniomandibular mechanics of being human. Proc. Royal Soc. London B 277, 3579–3586. http://dx.doi.org/10.1098/rspb.2010.0509.
Zysset, P.K., Edward GUO, X., Edward Hoffler, C., Moore, K.E., Goldstein, S.A., 1999. Elastic modulus and hardness of cortical and trabecular bone lamellae measured by nanoindentation in the human femur. J. Biomechan. 32, 1005–1012. http://dx.doi.org/10.1016/S0021-9290(99)00111-6.

Biocompatibility of fiber-reinforced composites for dental applications

3

A. Ballo[1] and T. Närhi[2,3]
[1]University of British Columbia, Vancouver, BC, Canada; [2]University of Turku, Turku, Finland; [3]Turku University Central Hospital, Turku, Finland

Abstract

Fiber-reinforced composites (FRCs) are a group of nonmetallic biomaterials that are growing in popularity in several dental applications. FRCs are a combination of two materials in which one of the materials, called the reinforcing phase, is in the form of fibers, and is embedded in the other material, called the matrix phase.

FRCs offers clinicians a material that can be tailored to mimic the properties of dentine or bone, to ensure good esthetic characters and to chemically bond to tooth structure. Interface properties are critical to the performance of FRCs because high masticatory forces are transferred across this interface. The most commonly used applications of FRCs are in removable dentures, minimally invasive fixed dental prostheses, periodontal splints, root canal posts, and orthodontic retainers.

This chapter is a broad overview of the biocompatibility of FRC materials currently used in dentistry. It also provides information on the biological aspects of FRC implants in cell culture conditions and in vivo. Clinical considerations are discussed based on current knowledge of use of polymers in regenerative medicine.

Chapter Outline

Biocompatibility of Dental Biomaterials. DOI: http://dx.doi.org/10.1016/B978-0-08-100884-3.00003-5

3.1 Introduction

Fiber-reinforced composites (FRCs) have gained widespread acceptance in a diverse range of structural engineering applications due to the development of materials with varying properties. Nowadays, FRCs are used in many structures, ranging from spacecraft and aircraft to buildings and bridges. FRCs have been applied in construction industries, decking, window and door frames, sports equipment, electronics, and medical applications (Mallick, 2008). FRCs are a relatively new group of materials among those that have traditionally been used in dental or medical applications over the last 40 years (Smith, 1961).

FRCs are durable materials with a lower elastic modulus than metals (Cheal et al., 1992). In fact, the mechanical strength and modulus of elasticity of unidirectional FRC (20–40GPa) are close to that of dentin and natural bone (Goldberg and Burstone, 1992). Therefore, it is not surprising that FRCs have the potential for use in many applications in dentistry such as periodontal splinting, orthodontic retention, root canal posts, reinforcement and repair of removable dentures as well as of fixed prostheses (Duncan et al., 2000; Freilich et al., 2002a,b,c; Freilich and Meiers, 2004). There is growing interest in using FRCs in oral implant applications and surgical implants for orthopedic and craniofacial surgery involving some degree of structural performance under load-bearing conditions (Ballo et al., 2014; Vallittu et al., 2015; Piitulainen et al., 2015).

FRCs are a combination of two materials in which one of the materials, called the reinforcing phase, is in the form of fibers, and is embedded in the other material called the matrix phase (Bunsell and Renard, 2005). The role of the fibers in a composite material is primarily of increasing the strength and stiffness of the simple resin system, while the resin bonds the fibers together and protects them from the external environment moisture (Vallittu, 1996).

FRCs have favorable mechanical properties, and their strength-to-weight ratios are superior to those of most alloys and offer other advantages, including being corrosion resistant, having a degree of translucency, and being relatively easily bonded to other materials and repaired. Additionally, FRCs provide alternatives for both chairside and laboratory fabrication.

FRCs can be classified according to the reinforcement and polymer matrices used. Glass fibers are the most commonly used reinforcing fibers in dental applications. Carbon/graphite, aramid, boron, and metal fibers have also been used (Edwards, 1998; Arhun and Arman, 2008). All of the different fibers used in composites have specific properties and so influence the overall behavior of the composite. To clearly describe an FRC it is also necessary to specify the geometry of the reinforcement, its concentration, distribution, and orientation (Alexander, 1996).

Several factors affect the strength of FRC materials, including the orientation and quantity of fibers, the impregnation and adhesion of fibers within the matrix polymer, as well as the properties of fibers versus the properties of the matrix polymer.

Fibers are mechanically more effective in achieving a durable and stiff composite than particulate fillers. The load-bearing capacity of the material can be increased with the aid of fibers (Fig. 3.1). However, the loading and direction of the fibers

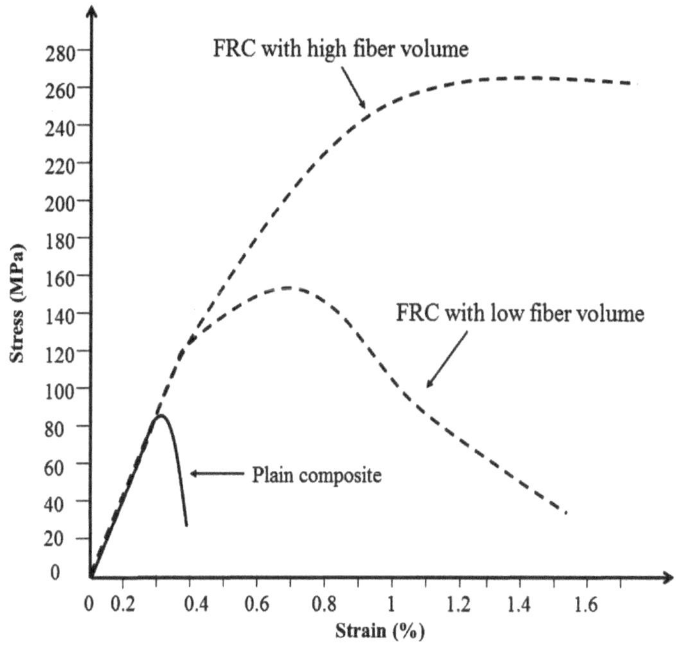

Figure 3.1 Typical stress–strain curves for fiber-reinforced composite.

influences the stiffness and strength of the composite. A unidirectional FRC has relative strength and stiffness comparable with metal when loading is directed along the fibers, but with much less weight. As a consequence of the anisotropic nature of unidirectional FRCs, the material has different physical properties in different directions. For this reason, the designing of an FRC prosthesis should be undertaken carefully. This is especially important in the oral environment as the prosthesis can experience varying mechanical loading in different directions. The use of woven fibers makes it possible to increase stiffness and strength in several directions.

3.2 Structure of fiber-reinforced composite

3.2.1 The matrix

The FRC has an interpenetrating polymer network (IPN) structure, where the matrix consists of a cross-linking polymer, a linear polymer, and a photoinitiator for inducing the polymerization reaction (Zhang and Matinlinna, 2011).

The mechanical strength of FRCs depends on the impregnation of fibers within the resin matrix and adhesion of fibers to the matrix (Vallittu, 1998, 1999). Setting reactions in the resin matrix are both polymerization reactions and cross-linking reactions. One of the most commonly used resin matrices, which form highly cross-linking polymer structures, is *bis*-phenol-A-diglycidylmethacrylate (*bis*-GMA) (Zhang and Matinlinna, 2011). Methyl methacrylate (MMA) a linear polymer (Zhang and Matinlinna, 2011) is joined to form a cross-linking polymer (Anusavice, 2009). The photoinitiator includes a photosensitizer and a reducing agent. Camphoroquinone (CQ) and *N-N*-cyanoethyl methylaniline (CEMA) are the commonly used photosensitizer and reducing agents (Zhang and Matinlinna, 2011).

A polymerization reaction is the formation of a polymer by sequential addition of monomeric units. Typical polymerization reactions are an addition (including free-radical addition polymerization) and condensation polymerizations (Darvell, 2006). The cross-linking reaction in a polymer refers to the formation of a cross-link where chains are bonded together either through a direct connection or an intermediary atom, ion, molecule, or chain.

3.2.2 Fiber composition

Fiberglass refers to a group of products made from individual glass fibers combined into a variety of forms. E-glass is one of the most attractive reinforcements due to its high performance, good combinations of chemical resistance and mechanical properties, and low cost. The composition of E-glass fiber is: 55% SiO_2, 22% CaO, 15% Al_2O_3, 6% B_2O_3, and 0.5% MgO. In addition, there are also small amounts (less than 1.0 wt%) of other metal oxides (Fe, Na, K). Glass fibers offer high tensile strength, excellent compression and impact properties, decent elastic modulus, good resistance to high temperatures and corrosive environments, and also superior esthetic appearance compared to carbon fibers.

Glass fibers can be divided into two major groups, according to their geometry: continuous (long) fibers and the discontinuous (short) fibers. The primary function of the fibers is to carry the loads along their longitudinal directions. The fiber orientation, content, distribution and the ability to maintain these parameters are significant for the reinforcement and thereby clinical success.

The fiber's type, length, orientation, and volume influence the following properties of the FRC (Soares et al., 1999): tensile strength and modulus, compressive strength and modulus, fatigue strength and fatigue failure mechanism, density, electrical and thermal conductivity, and finally their cost.

Unidirectional glass fibers are fiber rovings consisting of 1000–200,000 single glass fibers, depending on volume. Unidirectional fibers give anisotropic mechanical properties to the composite and are suitable for applications in which the direction of highest stress is known. Fibers woven in two directions (bidirectional fibers) reinforce construction in several directions, and are therefore useful when it is difficult to predict the direction of highest stress in the application.

3.2.3 Adhesion between fiber and matrix

The performance of FRCs is controlled by the properties of the fiber–matrix interface. Good adhesion between the fibers and the matrix is a primary requirement for effective use of reinforcement properties. This interfacial bonding (or adhesion) results in efficient stress transfer from the continuous matrix to the dispersed fiber reinforcement and can increase its ability to absorb energy (Reibhart and Clements, 1987). However, if the adhesion is not durable and if any voids appear between the fiber and the matrix, these voids may act as initial fracture sites in the composite and provoke the breakdown of the material (Thwe and Liao, 2002). Given this, durable adhesion between the fiber and the matrix is significant for the mechanical performance and the longevity of restoration in dental applications (De Vekey and Majumdar, 1970).

Treatment of the fibers is beneficial in order to improve the water resistance of fibers, enhance the wettability of fiber surface by resin, and promote interfacial adhesion. A coupling agent is a chemical that functions at the interface to create a chemical bridge between the reinforcement and matrix.

Silanes are recognized as efficient coupling agents extensively used in composites and adhesive formulations (Rider and Arnott, 2000). Silanes are hybrid inorganic–organic chemical compounds in which a carbon is directly attached to silicon. These compounds are silicon esters and are used as coupling agents in silanization treatment, sometimes called a silanation. This refers to the surface treatment aiming at promotion of bonding dissimilar matrices together (Matinlinna et al., 2004; Matinlinna and Vallittu, 2007).

Effective wetting of fibers by resin matrix, also called resin impregnation, is a prerequisite for their effective use before further steps in the fabrication of the final restoration in dentistry (Matinlinna and Vallittu, 2007). One current fiber reinforcement system based on preimpregnation utilizes highly porous linear polymers to preimpregnate the fibers. As a concept, an IPN is a combination of two or more polymers in network form that are synthesized in juxtaposition. They differ from polymer blends which are rougher in structure, and also differ from copolymers which are based on chemical reactions of monomer units and polymer backbones (Sperling, 1994). Currently in dental materials, IPN-like nanostructures are formed and used in denture base polymers, denture teeth and FRCs, and very recently in some novel restorative composite resins. In adhesive interfaces, IPN polymers and composites provide good adhesion to resin composites based on the secondary-IPN bonding due to swelling of the IPN nanostructure. Several adhesive interfaces between natural and synthetic biomaterials and adhesive resins by means of primers or coupling agents can also be considered as IPNs.

3.3 Clinical applications of fiber-reinforced composites in dentistry

The use of fiber-reinforced technology in dentistry dates back to the 1960s. Early attempts to adapt the technology for dental applications involved the incorporation of reinforcing fibers into polymethyl methacrylate (PMMA) denture base resin to reduce the incidence of fracture. Once resin-based composites became established as a restorative material in dentistry, attempts were made to use fiber reinforcement technology to provide sufficient strength for use as a fixed bridge.Currently, FRC

Table 3.1 **Clinical application of fiber-reinforced composites in dentistry**

Clinical application

• Reinforced direct composite restoration
• Root canal posts
• Single indirect restorations
  ◦ Inlay
  ◦ Onlay
  ◦ Partial/full veneer crowns
• Teeth splinting
  ◦ Periodontal splinting
  ◦ Post trauma splints
• Fixed dental prostheses (anterior and posterior)
  ◦ Simple cantilever
  ◦ Fixed-fixed
  ◦ Implant supported
• Immediate replacement transitional and long-term provisional bridges
• Reinforced or repairing dentures
• Fixed orthodontic retainers

materials have many applications in dental practice (Table 3.1). The potential advantages, as well as disadvantages of this group of materials, are listed in Table 3.2. The development of FRCs with a new type of resin system, combined with a better understanding of the design principles governing device construction, has led to the use of FRCs in a variety of disciplines and applications: removable prosthodontics, fixed prosthodontics, restorative dentistry, periodontology, orthodontics, and in repairs of fractured porcelain veneers (Vallittu, 2013). In general, the clinical uses of FRC fall into two categories: direct and indirect restorations. FRCs can be used to produce definitive fixed dental prostheses (FDPs) (Kangasniemi et al., 2003). Based on current clinical results, it is reasonable to expect FRC FDPs to attain a longevity of 10 years (Kangasniemi et al., 2003). FDPs made from FRC are classified in several different categories: surface-retained FDPs, inlay/onlay retained FDPs, full coverage crown and hybrid FPDs. FRC FDPs were usually reinforced with preimpregnated long fibers that are oriented mesio-distally in the main framework of an FRC FPD, and a hybrid particulate composite veneer. Since the substructure occupied a sufficiently large volume, the FDPs could serve for up to 4 or more years (Freilich et al., 2002a,b,c). According to a published clinical report, FRC FDPs could serve for 5–10 years (Feinman and Smidt, 1997). Moreover, FRCs have become a choice of material for immediate tooth replacement because of the convenience of this technique, which can be carried out at the dentist's office (Kermanshah and Motevasselian, 2010).

The use of FRCs in root canal posts to anchor cores and crowns has rapidly increased (Mannocci et al., 2005a,b,1999; Vallittu, 2013). FRC posts consist of a resin matrix, in which structural reinforced carbon fibers or quartz/glass fibers are

Table 3.2 Advantages and disadvantages of fiber-reinforced composites in dentistry

Advantages	Disadvantages
• Metal-free restoration • Single-visit immediate tooth replacements • Lower treatment costs • Suitable for transitional and long-term provisional restoration • Easily repaired • Good esthetics • Suitable for young patients (developing dentition) and old adults (time saving) • Simple production in laboratory without the need for waxing, investing and casting • Very conservative with minimal or no tooth preparation • Wear to opposing teeth much reduced in comparison to traditional metal-ceramic restorations	• Potential wear or chipping of the overlying composite especially in patients with parafunction • May lack sufficient rigidity for long span fixed dental prostheses • Careful moisture control is required for adhesive technique • Uncertain longevity in comparison to traditional techniques

embedded. Black carbon FRC posts are poorly suited for combination with translucent full ceramic restoration due to their unfavorable optical properties in comparison with the nearly tooth-colored quartz fiber and glass FRC posts. Glass FRCs can be used in root canals as both prefabricated solid posts and individually formed posts (Vallittu, 2013). Individually formed posts are made from nonpolymerized fiber-resin prepregs, typically consisting of glass fibers and light-curing matrix.

FRCs can also be used for periodontal splinting and stabilization of tooth mobility (Miller, 1993; Strassler et al., 1999; Strassler and Serio, 2007). There is no doubt that splinting does reduce tooth mobility while the splint is in place (Laudenbach et al., 1977). In the last decade, research supports the use of periodontal splinting as recommended therapy to stabilize those teeth to improve long-term prognosis (Wheeler et al., 1994; McGuire and Nunn, 1996; Bernal et al., 2002). In a long-term clinical evaluation of splinting over a period of 48–96 months, FRCs have been found to be very successful (Strassler et al., 2001). The success of these splints can be attributed to close adaptation of the fiber to the tooth surface combined with cross-stabilization of the mobile teeth by placing adhesive composite resin on the facial surfaces (Strassler et al., 2003; Strassler and Brown, 2001). Splinting of traumatized teeth with FRCs and adhesive composite resin has also been reported (Yildirim et al., 2006; Rudo, 2000). In order to stabilize the traumatized tooth or teeth or for tooth stabilization after transplantation, the tooth must be allowed to have some movement which can be achieved with the use of FRCs (Trope, 1995; McDonald and Strassler, 1999).

3.4 Fiber-reinforced composite performance in the oral environment

The conditions in which FRCs have to perform can be divided into biochemical and mechanical components. The biological and chemical conditions in the oral cavity make it a particularly hostile environment by accelerating the hydrophilic degradation processes. These are mainly related to the water-absorption properties and hydrophilic nature of FRCs and can result in the breakdown of the bond between the fiber and the resin. The main reason for this breakdown is the silane coupling-agent degradation, which reduces the mechanical properties of the FRCs. Mastication or chewing produces stresses in the dental restorations which vary in magnitude considerably, depending on diet and on the position of the tooth. The mean maximal occlusal forces in the incisal area have been reported to range from 264N to 370N (Laurell, 1985; Paphangkorakit and Osbom, 1997). In the molar region the forces can be around 800N (Van Eijden, 1991). Therefore, FRCs have to withstand a large number of cyclic stresses since fatigue-related mechanisms are constantly related in FRC restorations. According to a DIN standard, a FDP should withstand more than 1000N occlusal force in a static fracture resistance test. The maximum occlusal force may be applied 3000 times per day. Combining all these considerations together, FDP has to meet substantial cyclic loads over a long period of time in everyday use (Vallittu, 2001).

The loading-bearing capacity of FRC FDPs is higher than the maximum biting forces in the molar region (Ozcan et al., 2005; Dyer et al., 2005). In the FRC FDPs, the framework between the abutments is made of continuous unidirectional fibers in the mesio-distal direction, which offer high flexural strength (Vallittu, 1998; Nohrström et al., 2000). Clinical studies have shown that the FRC framework needs to provide support for the veneering composite resin and, therefore, additional fibers need to be placed inside the pontic (Freilich et al., 2002a,b,c). These can be reinforced with woven fibers. Whereas surface-retained FRC FDPs can be supported and bonded from both ends because of the flexibility of the FRC framework, the surface-retained resin-bonded FDPs made of metal are normally supported from one end only in order to avoid debonding. The flexibility of FRCs allows movement of abutment teeth to occur to some extent without compromising the prostheses. In the surface-retained FRC FDPs, the location of the bonding wing in the vertical dimension of the abutments is important. The fibers of the bonding wing should be placed as close as possible to the incisal edge to diminish the bending dislodgement forces.

FRCs have high tensile strength (700–1000 MPa) and at the same time, exhibit elasticity characteristics that are similar to dentin (Pfeiffer et al., 2002). This minimizes the risk of root fractures when using FRC posts, which are typically caused by tension peaks induced through loading and shear forces. The even load distribution is supported through the friction-locked bond between post and tooth substance, due to the adhesive luting of the FRC post.

Recent laboratory investigations have suggested that the failure forces of the experimental FRC specimens with an average dental implant diameter exceeded the reported maximum static human bite forces (Ballo et al., 2008a).

3.5 Biocompatibility and toxicity

Resin-based dental restorative materials are extensively used in dentistry today. However, significant concerns still remain regarding their biocompatibility (Soderholm and Marioti, 1999; Gosavi et al., 2010).

The residual monomers may influence the biocompatibility of FRCs (MacDougall et al., 1998), and cause some adverse biological reactions which can take place either locally or far from the site of contact (i.e., systemically). The latter is a very important consideration because it may not always be readily apparent that clinical symptoms such as dermatological, rheumatic or neural reactions could be associated with a biomaterial (Gosavi et al., 2010). Both patients and the dental personnel are exposed to these interactions and the potential risks, with the patient being the recipient of the restorative materials and the dental personnel handling many materials on a daily basis. The "no-touch" technique, i.e., using gloves, may prevent materials' adverse effects for dental personnel.

Some released compounds may cause biological reactions (Soderholm and Marioti, 1999), and a case of contact allergy caused by *bis*-GMA has been reported (Stoeva et al., 2008). *Bis*-GMA has also been reported as the most cytotoxic monomer among dental resin composite monomers (Moharamzadeh et al., 2009), thus it is important that the FRC materials should have a high degree of monomer conversion. This can be obtained by increasing the photopolymerization time in combination with heat-induced postcuring (Ferracane and Condon, 1992).

In general, the initial resin monomers in FRC may reach a conversion rate between 35% and 77% through polymerization when light cured (Darvell, 2006). A degree of monomer conversion of approximately 90% can be achieved by photopolymerization in a vacuum and postcuring for 24 hours at 120°C (Ballo et al., 2008a).

3.5.1 Cellular responses

Several cell culture methods and cell types have been used to determine the cytotoxicity and in vitro biocompatibility of FRCs. These studies have demonstrated that most of the components of the resin composites are toxic in direct contact with fibroblasts (Schedle et al., 1998; Schmalz, 1998; Wataha et al., 1994). According to Yoshii (1997), clear relationships between monomer structures and cytotoxicity are apparent. In general, acrylates are more toxic than methacrylates, and a hydroxyl group within the monomer enhances the cytotoxicity. The dimethacrylates, such as 2,2-*bis* [4-(2-hydroxy-3-methacryloyloxy-propyloxy)phenyl-] propane, also known as *bis*-GMA, and urethane dimethacrylate (UDMA) had stronger toxic effects than monomethacrylates and 7 *bis*-GMA is more toxic than UDMA (Yoshii, 1997).

Vallittu and Ekstrand (1999) studied fiber-reinforced dental materials (fiber-reinforced poly(methyl methacrylate) composites) and reported no cytotoxicity. In addition, some long-term cytotoxicity studies have been carried out for dental restorative materials containing different dimethacrylates which have found that materials become less cytotoxic after aging (Bouillaguet et al., 2002).

Ferracane et al. (1998) found that the poor curing significantly affects the mechanical properties of the restoration material. In addition, the release of residual monomers from *bis*-GMA–TEGDMA polymer might influence the biocompatibility of the restoration material (MacDougall et al., 1998). As a result of this, composite implants should have an optimum degree of monomer conversion. The main factors affecting the degree of monomer conversion are, of course, the curing time and intensity, as well as the distance of the light-curing device from the material surface (Leloup et al., 2002). The optimum degree of monomer conversion can be obtained by lengthening the photopolymerization time in combination with postpolymerization at increased temperature (Ferracane and Condon, 1992). Ballo et al. (2008a) have shown that a degree of monomer conversion of approximately 90% of the polymer can be achieved by photopolymerization followed by postcuring for 24 hours at 120°C. With further storage in water, the residual monomers are leached out from the composite implants (Ballo et al., 2008b).

According to Säilynoja et al. (2004), in cell culture conditions only small changes in fibroblast morphology were observed after the light and 15-minute heat polymerization compared with negative controls during the 24 hours observation period.

According to Abdulmajeed et al. (2014), an FRC surface enhances blood clotting time compared with a plain polymer surface. Platelet adhesion and activation are crucial events in wound healing as they influence the subsequent formation of thrombus. The reason for enhanced blood clotting and higher platelet activity is probably due to the higher surface free energy (SFE) of the FRC substrates because it is well known that there is a complex dependence between platelet adhesion and surface wettability and energy (Abdulmajeed et al., 2014). Abdulmajeed et al. (2014) also reported higher resistance to enzymatic detachment of human gingival fibroblasts over 24-hour incubation on FRC substrates compared with plain polymer. This can be related to the differences in surface properties of the materials. The better resistance of fibroblasts on FRC substrates against enzymatic detachment is probably related to the high SFE that is known to have strong influence on wetting, adsorption, and cell adhesion behaviors (Ponsonnet et al., 2003).

The proliferation and osteogenic potential of bone-marrow-derived osteoblast-like cells have been investigated on FRC substrates (Ballo et al., 2008b). It was observed that osteoblast attachment, proliferation and differentiation on the *bis*-GMA-TEGMA polymer with E-glass fiber reinforcement was comparable with that observed on a grit-blasted titanium surface over a 21-day cell culture period. A scanning electron microscopy (SEM) investigation revealed that cultured cells proliferated on all experimental FRC surfaces and eventually formed multicellular layers that entirely covered the specimens. After 21 days of culture, no visible differences could be noted between different FRC substrates and titanium, indicating that the tested FRC specimens were cytocompatible, with a similar cellular response to that observed on titanium.

Ballo (2008) examined experimental bioactive FRC implants which contained biostable organic polymers and glass fibers, with surface modification of bioactive glass (BAG) particles. BAG was thought to enhance bone formation on FRC implants (Ballo et al., 2008b). The bone-marrow-derived osteoblast-like cells seeded on FRC-BAG substrates have been shown to stop proliferating when their alkaline phosphatase

(ALP) activity reaches a peak value during the second week of culture (Ballo et al., 2008b). Furthermore, their gene expression profiles (osteocalcin and bone sialoprotein) increased to levels similar to those on the titanium surface and the cells started to mineralize extracellular matrix more rapidly than the cells seeded on titanium. The enhanced differentiation cascade with FRC-BAG was probably related to Ca, PO_4, and Si ions initially released from the BAG (Hench et al., 2004; Radin et al., 2005; Vallittu et al., 2015). The Ca and Si ions released from the BAG are known to enhance maturation of bone-forming cells (Yao et al., 2005). Hench and West (1996) proposed that the release of soluble silica from the surface of BAGs might be at least partially responsible for stimulating the proliferation of bone-forming cells on BAG surfaces.

3.5.2 *In vivo behavior*

In a series of in vivo studies (Ballo, 2008; Ballo et al., 2009, 2011, 2014), FRC implants exhibited sufficient flexural strength to resist fracture under loading conditions exceeding reported maximum static human bite forces, and in a bone environment induce neither toxic nor inflammatory reactions.

Residual methyl methacrylate monomers (MMA) leaching from PMMA-based FRCs have even been associated with cytotoxic effects, but this has been proven to be clinically irrelevant after adequate processing and preoperative storage (Vallittu et al., 1995; Miettinen and Vallittu, 1997). Based on histological and SEM observations, the porous surface structure of FRC implants enhances appositional bone growth on the implant surface (Fig. 3.2) (Ballo et al., 2009, 2011, 2014). Under load-bearing conditions, the implant appears to function like an osteoconductive prosthesis, enabling direct mobilization and rapid return to full weight-bearing condition (Hautamäki et al., 2008). It has been shown in experimental animals that the polymer surface can guarantee equal bone bonding volume after 4 and 12 weeks of healing with titanium (Ballo et al., 2009, 2014). Neither grit-blasted FRC implants nor BAG-coated FRC implants showed adverse reactions to the pig bone tissue during the 12-week healing period (Ballo et al., 2009). The immediate close contact of osseous tissue to the bis-GMA-TEGMA polymer with E-glass fiber reinforcement indicated that the FRC implants have appropriate host contact in the bone environment (Vallittu et al., 2015).

Thus, the surface modification of FRC implants with BAG particles significantly increases the bone bonding area and increases the bonding strength of FRC implants to the bone when compared with FRC implants without BAG (Ballo et al., 2009, 2011). In the histological evaluations bone has been found to be in direct contact with exposed BAG particles in different experimental conditions (Vallittu et al., 2015).

3.6 Conclusion

FRCs have been introduced in a variety of clinical applications. Currently, continuous unidirectional glass FRCs provide the highest strength and are the most appropriate for dental use. Several parameters, including the fiber volume and fiber direction, have a substantial impact on the mechanical properties of FRC materials. An appreciation of

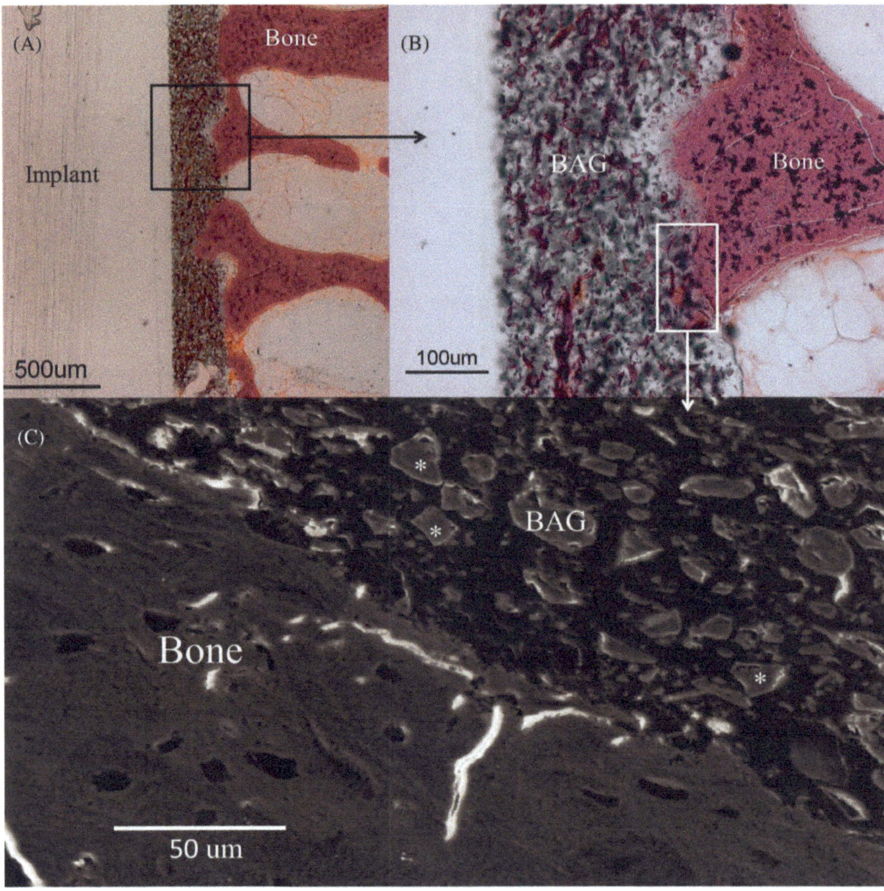

Figure 3.2 Histological non-decalcified ground and SEM sections of bone contact on FRC–BAG implants. (A) Low-magnification image shows a large volume of newly formed bone growing directly and along the implant surface. (B) Higher magnification of image (A). (C) SEM image shows the newly formed bone is in direct contact with the BAG coating and adapted perfectly to the microirregularities and porosities of the implant surface.

the critical factors which impact on the properties and clinical service potential of FRC restorations will assist the practitioner and dental technician in designing and delivering high-quality restorations, which will maximize the success rate and longevity of these new materials.

FRC prostheses offer the advantages of good esthetics, minimally invasive treatment, and an ability to bond to the abutment teeth, thereby compensating for less than optimal abutment tooth retention and resistance form.

Recent experimental animal studies have shown that the FRC implants with a BAG surface layer establish equal osseointegration with the titanium implants with similar surface texture. It is likely that research with new materials not yet used in biomedical applications will further extend the potential of FRC materials.

References

Abdulmajeed, A.A., Walboomers, X.F., Massera, J., Kokkari, A.K., Vallittu, P.K., Närhi, T.O., 2014. Blood and fibroblast responses to thermoset BisGMA-TEGDMA/glass fiber-reinforced composite implants in vitro. Clin. Oral Implants Res. 25 (7), 843–851.

Anusavice, K.J., 2009., 11th ed Phillip's Science of Dental Materials, 2009 Elsevier Science, St. Louis, MO, 77.

Arhun, N., Arman, A., 2008. Fiber-reinforced technology in multidisciplinary chairside approaches. Indian J. Dent. Res. 19 (3), 272–277.

Ballo, A.M., 2008. Fiber-reinforced composite as oral implant material, experimental studies of glass fiber and bioactive glass in vitro and in vivo. Annales Universitatis Turkensis.

Ballo, A.M., Lassila, L.V., Vallittu, P.K., Närhi, T.O., 2007. Load bearing capacity of bone anchored fiber-reinforced composite device. J. Mater. Sci. 18 (10), 2025–2031.

Ballo, A.M., Lassila, L.V., Vallittu, P.K., Närhi, T.O., 2008a. In vitro mechanical testing of glass fiber-reinforced composite as dental implants. J. Contemp. Dent. Pract. 9 (2), 41–48.

Ballo, A.M., Kokkari, A.K., Meretoja, V.V., Lassila, L.V., Vallittu, P.K., Närhi, T.O., 2008b. Osteoblast proliferation and maturation on bioactive fiber-reinforced composite surface. J. Mater. Sci. 19 (10), 3169–3177.

Ballo, A.M., Akca, E.A., Ozen, T., Lassila, L., Vallittu, P.K., Närhi, T.O., 2009. Bone tissue responses to glass fiber-reinforced composite implants—a histomorphometric study. Clin. Oral Implants Res. 20 (6), 608–615.

Ballo, A.M., Närhi, T.O., Akca, E.A., Ozen, T., Lassila, L., Syrjänen, S.M., et al., 2011. Prepolymerized vs. in situ polymerized fiber-reinforced composite implants—a pilot study. J. Dent. Res. 90 (2), 263–267.

Ballo, A.M., Cekic-Nagas, I., Ergun, G., Lassila, L., Palmquist, A., Thomsen, P., et al., 2014. Osseointegration of fiber-reinforced composite implants: a histological and ultrastructural observation. Dent. Mater. 30 (12), 384–395.

Bernal, G., Carvajal, J.C., Munoz-Viveros, C.A., 2002. A review of the clinical management of mobile teeth. J. Contemp. Dent. Pract. 3 (4), 10–22.

Bouillaguet, S., Shaw, L., Gonzalez, L., Wataha, J.C., Krejci, I., 2002. Long-term cytotoxicity of resin-based dental restorative materials. J. Oral Rehabil. 29 (1), 7–13.

Bunsell, A.R., Renard, J., 2005. Fundamentals of Fibre Reinforced Composite Materials. Institute of Physics Publishing, Bristol, MA.

Cheal, E.J., Spector, M., Hayes, W.C., 1992. Role of loads and prosthesis material properties on the mechanics of the proximal femur after total hip arthroplasty. J. Orthop. Res. 10 (3), 405–422.

Darvell, B.W., 2006. In: Darvell, B.W. (Ed.), Materials Science for Dentistry, 8th edn. Woodhead, Pokfulam.

De Vekey, R.C., Majumdar, A.J., 1970. Interfacial bond strength of glass fibre reinforced cement composites. J. Mater. Sci. 5(Letters), 183–185.

Duncan, J.P., Freilich, M.A., Latvis, C.J., 2000. Fiber-reinforced composite framework for implant supported overdentures. J. Prosthet. Dent. 84 (2), 200–204.

Edwards, K.L., 1998. An overview of the technology of fiber-rinforced plastics for design purposes. Mater. Des. 19 (1), 1–10.

Feinman, R.A., Smidt, A., 1997. A combination porcelain/fiber-reinforced composite bridge: a case report. Pract. Periodontics Aesthet. Dent. 9 (8), 925–929.
Ferracane, L., Condon, J.R., 1992. Post-cure heat treatments for composites: properties and fractography. Dent. Mater. 8 (5), 290–295.
Ferracane, J.L., Berge, H.X., Condon, J.R., 1998. In vitro aging of dental composites in water: effect of degree of conversion, filler volume, and filler/matrix coupling. J. Biomed. Mater. Res. 42 (3), 465–472.
Freilich, M.A., Meiers, J.S., 2004. Fiber-reinforced composite prostheses. Dent. Clin. North. Am. 48 (2), 545–562.
Freilich, M.A., Duncan, J.P., Alarcon, E.K., Eckrote, K.A., 2002a. The design and fabrication of fiberreinforced implant prostheses. J. Prosthet. Dent. 88 (4), 449–454.
Freilich, M.A., Meiers, J.C., Duncan, J.P., Eckrote, K.A., Goldberg, A.J., 2002b. Clinical evaluation of fiber-reinforced fixed bridges. J. Am. Dent. Assoc. 133 (11), 1524–1534.
Freilich, M.A., Meiers, J.C., Duncan, J.P., Eckrote, K.A., Goldberg, A.J., 2002c. JADA Continuing Education. American Dental Association, Chicago, IL.
Goldberg, A.J., Burstone, C.J., 1992. The use of continuous fiber reinforcement in dentistry. Dent. Mater. 8 (3), 197–202.
Gosavi, S.S., Gosavi, S.Y., Alla, R.K., 2010. Local and systemic effects of unpolymerised monomers. Dent. Res. J. (Isfahan) 7 (2), 82–87.
Hautamäki, M.P., Aho, A.J., Alander, P., Rekola, J., Gunn, J., Strandberg, N., et al., 2008. Repair of bone segment defects with surface porous fiber-reinforced polymethyl methacrylate (PMMA) composite prosthesis: histomorphometric incorporation model and characterization by SEM. Acta. Orthop. 79 (4), 555–564.
Hench, L.L., West, J.K., 1996. In Life Chemistry Reports. Harwood Academic Publishers, Amsterdam, 178.
Hench, L.L., Xynos, I.D., Polak, J.M., 2004. Bioactive glasses for in situ tissue regeneration. J. Biomater. Sci. Polym. Ed. 15 (4), 543–562.
Kangasniemi, I., Vallittu, P.K., Meiers, J., Dyer, S.R., Rosentritt, M., 2003. Consensus statement on fiber-reinforced polymers: current status, future directions, and how they can be used to enhance dental care. Int. J. Prosthodont. 16 (2), 209.
Kermanshah, H., Motevasselian, F., 2010. Immediate tooth replacement using fiber-reinforced composite and natural tooth pontic. Oper. Dent. 35 (2), 238–245.
Laudenbach, K.W., Stoller, N., Laster, L., 1977. The effects of periodontal surgery on horizontal tooth mobility. J. Dent. Res. 56 (Special Issue) abstract no. 596.
Laurell, L., 1985. Occlusal forces and chewing ability in dentitions with cross-arch bridges. Swed. Dent. J. Suppl. 26, 160–167.
Leloup, G., Holvoet, P.E., Bebelman, S., Devaux, J., 2002. Raman scattering determination of the depth of cure of light-activated compoisites: influence of different clinically relevant paramaters. J. Oral Rehabil. 29 (6), 510–515.
MacDougall, M., Selden, J.K., Nydegger, J.R., Carnes, D.L., 1998. Immortalized mouse odontoblast cell line MO6-G3application G3application for in vitro biocompatibility testing. Am. J. Dent. 11, 11–16.
Mallick, P.K., 2008. Fiber-Reinforced Composites: Materials, Manufacturing, and Design, 3rd edn CRC Press, Taylor & Francis Group, Boca Raton, FL.
Mannocci, F., Ferrari, M., Watson, T.F., 1999. Intermittent loading of teeth restored using quartz fiber, carbon-quartz fiber, and zirconium dioxide ceramic root canal posts. J. Adhes. Dent. 1 (2), 153–158.
Mannocci, F., Qualtrough, A.J., Worthington, H.V., Watson, T.F., Pitt Ford, T.R., 2005a. Randomized clinical comparison of endodontically treated teeth restored with amalgam or with fiber posts and resin composite: five-year results. Oper. Dent. 30 (1), 9–15.

Mannocci, F., Sherriff, M., Watson, T.F., Vallittu, P.K., 2005b. Penetration of bonding resins into fibre-reinforced composite posts: a confocal microscopic study. Int. Endod. J. 38 (1), 46–51.
Matinlinna, J.P., Vallittu, P.K., 2007. Bonding of resin composites to etchable ceramic surfaces - an insight review of the chemical aspects on surface conditioning. J. Oral Rehabil. 34 (8), 622.
Matinlinna, J.P., Lassila, L.V.J., Özcan, M., Yli-Urpo, A., Vallittu, P.K., 2004. An introduction to silanes and their clinical applications in dentistry. Int. J. Prosthod. 17 (2), 155–164.
McDonald, N., Strassler, H.E., 1999. Evaluation for tooth stabilization and treatment of traumatized teeth. Dent. Clin. North Am. 43 (1), 135–149.
McGuire, M.K., Nunn, M.E., 1996. Prognosis versus actual outcome. II. The effectiveness of clinical parameters in developing an accurate diagnosis. J. Periodontol. 67 (1), 666–674.
Miller, T.E., 1993. A new material for periodontal splinting and orthodontic retention. Compend. Continu. Educat. Dent. 14 (6), 800–806.
Moharamzadeh, K., Brook, I.M., Van Noort, R., 2009. Biocompatibility of resin-based dental materials. Materials 2 (2), 514–548.
Nohrström, T.J., Vallittu, P.K., Yli-Urpo, A., 2000. The effect of placement and quantity of glass fibers on the fracture resistance of interim fixed partial dentures. Int. J. Prosthod. 13 (1), 72–78.
Ozcan, M., Breuklander, M.H., Vallittu, P.K., 2005. The effect of box preparation on the strength of glass fiber-reinforced composite inlay-retained fixed partial dentures. J. Prosthet. Dent. 93 (4), 337–345.
Paphangkorakit, J., Osbom, J.W., 1997. The effect of pressure on maximum incisal bite force in man. Arch. Oral Biol. 42 (1), 11–17.
Pfeiffer, P., Nergiz, I., Platzer, U., 2002. Yield strength of zirconia and glass fiber-reinforced posts. J. Dent. Res. 81, 428–430.
Piitulainen, J.M., Posti, J.P., Aitasalo, K.M., Vuorinen, V., Vallittu, P.K., Serlo, W., 2015. Paediatric cranial defect reconstruction using bioactive fibre-reinforced composite implant: early outcomes. Acta Neurochirurgica (Wien) 157 (4), 681–687.
Ponsonnet, L., Reybier, K., Jaffrezic, N., Comte, V., Lagneau, C., Lissac, M., et al., 2003. Relationship between surface properties (roughness, wettability) of titanium and titanium alloys and cell behavior. Mater. Sci. Eng. C 23, 551–560.
Radin, S., Reilly, G., Bhargave, G., Leboy, P.S., Ducheyne, P., 2005. Osteogenic effects of bioactive glass on bone marrow stromal cells. J. Biomed. Mater. Res. A 73 (1), 21–29.
Reibhart, T.J., Clements, L.L., 1987. In Engineered Materials Handbook, 1. ASM International, Park, OH, 27–34
Rider, A.N., Arnott, D.R., 2000. Boiling water and silane pre-treatment of aluminium alloy for durable adhesive bonding. Int. J. Adhes. 20, 209–220.
Rudo, D.N., 2000. Treatment option for dentoalveolar trauma. Quintessence. Int. 31 (9), 610.
Säilynoja, E.S., Shinya, A., Koskinen, M.K., Salonen, J.I., Masuda, T., Shinya, A., et al., 2004. Heat curing of UTMA-based hybrid resin: effects on the degree of conversion and cytotoxicity. Odontology 92, 27–35.
Schedle, A., Franz, A., Rausch-Fan, X., Spitter, A., Lucas, T., Samorapoompichit, P., et al., 1998. Cytotoxicity effects of dental composites, adhesive substances, compomers and cements. Dent. Mater. 14 (6), 429–440.
Schmalz, G., Arenholt-Bindslev, D., 2009. Biocompatibility of Dental Materials. Springer, New York, NY.
Smith, D.C., 1961. The acrylic denture: mechanical evaluation of midline fracture. Br. Dent. J. 110, 257–267.
Soares, C.A.M., Soares, C.M.M., Freitas, M.J.M., 1999. Mechanics of Composite Materials and Structures. Springer, New York, NY.

Soderholm, K.J., Marioti, A., 1999. Bis-GMA based resins in dentistry: are they safe? J. Am. Dent. Assoc. 130 (2), 201–209.

Sperling, L.H., 1994. IPN around the world In: Klemper, D. Sperling, L.H. Utracki, L.A. (Eds.), Interpenetrating Polymer Networks, vol. 4. Technomic, Lancaster, PA, pp. 3–11.

Stoeva, I., Kisselova, A., Zekova, M., 2008. Allergic contact stomatitis from bisphenol-A-glycidil methacrylate during application of composite restorations. A case report. J. IMAB, Ann. Proc., 45–46. book 2.

Strassler, H.E., Brown, C., 2001. Periodontal splinting with a thin, high-modulus polyethylene ribbon. Compend. Continu. Educat. Dent. 22 (8), 696–704.

Strassler, H.E., Serio, C.L., 2007. Esthetic considerations when splinting with fiber-reinforced composites. Dent. Clin. North Am. 51 (2), 507–524.

Strassler, H.E., Haeri, A., Gultz, J.P., 1999. New generation bonded reinforcing materials for anterior periodontal tooth stabilization and splinting. Dent. Clin. North Am. 43 (1), 105–126.

Strassler, H.E., Karbhari, V., Rudo, D., 2001. Effect of fiber reinforcement on flexural strength of composite. J. Dent. Res. 80 (Special Issue), 221. (abstract no. 854).

Strassler, H.E., Tomona, N., Spitznagel Jr, J.K., 2003. Stablizing periodontally compromised teeth with fiber-reinforced composite resin. Dent. Today 22 (9), 102–109.

Thwe, M.M., Liao, K., 2002. Effects of environmental aging on the mechanical properties of bamboo/glass fiber reinforced polymer matrix hybrid composites. Compos. Part A 33 (1), 43.

Trope, M., 1995. Clinical management of the avulsed tooth. Dent. Clin. North Am. 39 (1), 93–112.

Vallittu, P.K., 1998. The effect of glass fiber reinforcement on the fracture resistance of provisional fixed partial denture. J. Prosth. Dent. 79 (2), 125–130.

Vallittu, P.K., 1999. Flexural properties of acrylic resin polymers reinforced with unidirectional and woven glass fibers. J. Prosth. Dent. 81 (3), 318–326.

Vallittu, P.K., 2001. The second international symposium on fiber-reinforced plastics in dentistry. University of Turku, Turku, Finland.

Vallittu, P.K., 2013. Fibre-reinforced composites (FRCs) as dental materials. In: Vallittu, P.K. (Ed.), Non-Metallic Biomaterials for Tooth Repair and Replacement. Woodhead Publishing, Oxford, pp. 352–374.

Vallittu, P., Ekstrand, K., 1999. In vitro cytotoxicity of fiber-polymethyl methacrylate composite used in dentures. J. Oral Rehabil. 26 (8), 666–671.

Vallittu, P.K., Sevelius, C., 2000. Resin-bonded, glass fiber-reinforced composite fixed partial dentures: a clinical study. J. Prosth. Dent. 84 (4), 413–418.

Vallittu, P.K., Närhi, T.O., Hupa, L., 2015. Fiber glass-bioactive glass composite for bone replacing and bone anchoring implants. Dent. Mater. 31 (4), 371–381.

Van Eijden, T.M., 1991. Three-dimensional analyses of human bite-force magnitude and moment. Arch. Oral Biol. 36 (7), 535–539.

Wataha, J.C., Hanks, C.T., Strawn, S.E., Fat, J.C., 1994. Cytotoxicity of components of resins and other dental restorative materials. J. Oral Rehabil. 21 (4), 453–462.

Wheeler, T.T., McArthur, W.P., Magnusson, I., Marks, R.G., Smith, J., Sarrett, D.C., et al., 1994. Modeling the relationship between clinical, microbiologic, and immunologic parameters and alveolar bone levels in an elderly population. J. Periodontol. 65 (1), 68–78.

Yao, J., Radin, S., Reilly, G., Leboy, P.S., Ducheyne, P., 2005. Solution-mediated effect of bioactive glass in poly (lactic-co-glycolic acid)-bioactive glass composites on osteogenesis of marrow stromal cells. J. Biomed. Mater. Res. A 75 (4), 794–801.

Yildirim, Oz. G., Ataoglu, H., Kir, N., Karaman, A.I., 2006. An alternative method for splinting of traumatized teeth: case reports. Dent. Traumatol. 22 (6), 345–349.
Yoshii, E., 1997. Cytotoxic effects of acrylates and methacrylates: relationships of monomer structures and cytotoxicity. J. Biomed. Mater. Res. 37 (4), 517–524.
Zhang, M., Matinlinna, J.P., 2011. The effect of resin matrix composition on mechanical properties of E-glass fibre-reinforced composite for dental use. J. Adhes. Sci. Technol. 19 (25), 2687–2701.

Biocompatibility of biomaterials for dental tissue repair

4

P. Murray
Nova Southeastern University College of Dental Medicine,
Fort Lauderdale, FL, United States

Abstract

All dentists and dental patients will benefit from the reduced health risks afforded by guiding dentists to select biomaterials demonstrating biocompatibility for dental tissue repair. Most dentists are concerned about the potential toxic effects of restorative dental biomaterials, and many dentists have had patients who refuse to allow amalgam restorations to be used to restore their teeth. The biocompatibility of dental repair biomaterials can vary greatly with the most toxic generally being zinc oxide eugenol (ZOE), and the least toxic being biomaterials formulated for vital pulp therapy, such as tri-calcium silicate cements (mineral trioxide aggregate (MTA)). The other types of biomaterials (glass ionomers, composite resins, adhesives, sealers, and amalgam) are less toxic than ZOE, but still do not demonstrate suitable biocompatibility to be placed in direct contact with vital tissues. During the past decade, MTA has replaced calcium hydroxide as the first choice of biomaterial for placing in contact with a vital pulp. MTA has low toxicity and good sealing properties to prevent microleakage. MTA can also stimulate the release of growth factors, which promotes the healing and repair of vital pulp tissues. Other biomaterials, such as Emdogain for periodontal regeneration, and PepGen P15 for bone augmentation, contain active growth factors to promote tissue regeneration. Successful dental repair materials must lack toxicity, demonstrate biocompatibility, not induce inflammation sensitivity or pain, be physically stable and seal to prevent bacterial microleakage, and promote tissue repair by creating an environment where growth factors can induce stem cells and local cells to heal injured tissues.

Chapter Outline

Biocompatibility of Dental Biomaterials. DOI: http://dx.doi.org/10.1016/B978-0-08-100884-3.00004-7

4.1 Introduction

The ideal biomaterial for dental tissue repair demonstrates biocompatibility, however there is no biomaterial which accomplishes this completely and often when a biomaterial is placed in contact with the vital dental pulp or other dental tissue some cell death and tissue injury is unavoidable (Murray et al., 2003). It has been estimated that one out of every four (22.5%) to one out of eight (12%) dental patients, will experience allergic sensitivity and healing complications attributable to the dental biomaterial used to restore their teeth (Mjor, 1992). Some of these adverse responses could have been prevented if the dental biomaterials demonstrating biocompatibility were used to restore teeth (Murray et al., 2007). Eighty-three percent (83%) of dentists do not believe that enough is known about the toxic effects of restorative dental materials, 76% of dentists believe that dental materials can temporarily or permanently poison a patient. Only 9% of dentists are aware that zinc oxide eugenol (ZOE) is the most toxic of all the restorative dental biomaterials (unpublished data). The biomaterials that are the most compatible with dental tissues are generally the most chemically stable and physically inert; this prevents the release and leaching of potentially toxic chemicals (Geurtsen, 2000). This explains why mineral trioxide aggregate (MTA) has replaced calcium hydroxide ($Ca(OH)_2$) as the first choice of biomaterial for placing in contact with a vital pulp by most dentists (Witherspoon, 2008).

4.2 Future trends

All dentists and dental patients will benefit from the reduced health risks afforded by selecting the biomaterials demonstrating biocompatibility for dental tissue repair. Over time, the definition of biocompatibility has changed from being simply a lack of toxicity (Cox et al., 1987), lack of cytotoxicity (Neupert and Welker, 1980), good tissue tolerance (Müller et al., 1990), lack of genotoxicity (Ribeiro et al., 2006), lack of mutagenicity (Kostoryz et al., 2003) to include favorable tissue healing and tissue regeneration (Murray et al., 2002a,b). The improvements in research design, increased clinical and scientific knowledge, and the use of new technology has improved our ability to formulate dental biomaterials demonstrating biocompatibility. The results of biocompatibility testing have shown that a common temporary restorative material, ZOE, is the most cytotoxic dental material (Hensten-Pettersen and Helgeland, 1977). So cytotoxic is ZOE that it has become the international standard for establishing the limit for acceptable biocompatibility, meaning that any biomaterial that is found to be more toxic than ZOE does not have an acceptable biocompatibility for clinical use (International Organization for Standardization 7405 and 10993). Most dental materials, including glass ionomers, composite resins, adhesives, sealers, and amalgam are less toxic than ZOE, but are still not suitable to be placed in direct contact with vital pulp, periodontal, or periapical tissues (Pameijer and Stanley, 1998). Biocompatibility testing has shown that the most toxic state of most dental materials is prior to setting or polymerization, when highly toxic nonpolymerized monomers can leach from the materials into adjacent pulp tissues.

The increasing focus of dentists on selecting the most appropriate biomaterials for placement in contact with vital tissues may be more advantageous to promote tissue healing and may be better at preventing potential health hazards, adverse events, allergic sensitivity, and treatment failure. This trend can be seen with the increasing replacement of $Ca(OH)_2$, as the former first choice of material for vital pulp therapy and root repair with alternative types of biomaterials. Today's most popular dental pulp capping and root repair materials have been formulated to demonstrate appropriate biocompatibility with dental tissues, thereby avoiding the necrosis sometimes seen when $Ca(OH)_2$ was placed in direct contact with a vital dental pulp (Turner et al., 1987). The latest biomaterials created specifically for direct pulp capping and root repair include tri-calcium silicate cements, such as ProRoot MTA, or Biodentine, and related bio-ceramic biomaterials, such as EndoSequence Root Repair Material (ESRRM). The success of the tri-calcium silicate cements and bioceramics was previously assumed to be because they were chemically stable and physically inert (Torabinejad et al., 1995), thereby avoiding the release and leaching of potentially toxic chemicals. This explains why the highly alkaline and soluble $Ca(OH)_2$ has been replaced by tri-calcium silicate cements (MTA or Biodentine) by most dentists for the direct capping of the vital pulp, periodontal, or periapical tissues. Recent studies indicate that the success of tri-calcium silicate cements may be partly because they can stimulate the release of growth factors in adjacent tissues and the growth factors found in dentine (Tomson et al., 2007), such as transforming growth factor $\beta 1$ (TGF-$\beta 1$) which can promote tissue healing and regeneration (Dobie et al., 2002). A promising area of research is the development of biomaterials, membranes, and scaffolds which release bioactive compounds, such as Emdogain (Abbas et al., 2003) to promote periodontal regeneration and P-15 to promote bone regeneration (Emam et al., 2011). The types and variety of bioactive dental biomaterials are expected to grow in the future, because of their ability to promote dental tissue regeneration above the normal level of healing. A schematic representation of the past, present, and future most popular biomaterials for dental tissue regeneration is shown in Fig. 4.1.

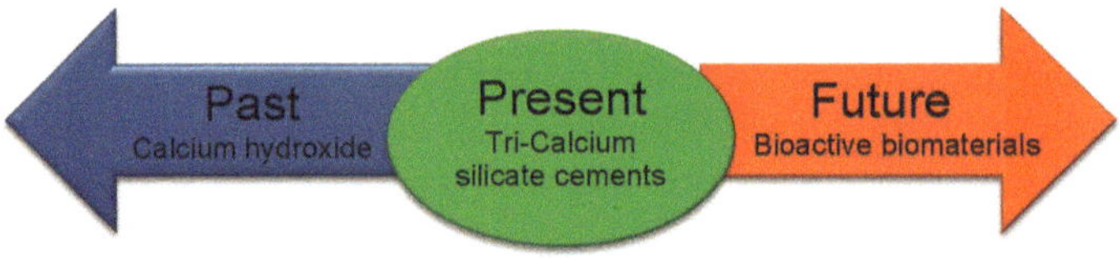

Figure 4.1 Past, present, and future most-popular biomaterials for dental pulp and periapical tissue regeneration.

4.3 Sources of further information and advice

Only a few of the dental biomaterials which are sold commercially have passed all the biocompatibility screening standards to ensure they have a very low toxicity, are safe, clinically effective, and beneficial for patients. Most dental biomaterials have not been tested for their biocompatibility, because they were approved using a grandfather process. The grandfather process allows the sale and marketing of biomaterials without any biocompatibility testing, provided the biomaterial has a similar chemical composition, sterilization, manufacturing process, and amount of body contact as a marketed biomaterial. In the rare event, where an entirely novel chemical formulation of biomaterial has been created, the US Food and Drug Administration (FDA) requires biological evaluation of medical devices submitted either for premarket notification via the 510(k) process or for premarket approval. The FDA has adopted the ISO-10993 standard criteria (Fig. 4.2) for guiding the selection of biocompatibility tests for a given type of device, which includes dental biomaterials.

The ISO standard lists recommended tests based on the type and duration of body contact. Guidance from the FDA in Memorandum #G95-1 stresses that while ISO 10993 should be used as a guide, some devices may require fewer or more tests than those that are indicated in ISO 10993, and manufacturers are encouraged to discuss testing plans with the appropriate FDA review division prior to initiation of testing. The phases of biocompatibility testing that apply to dental repair biomaterials are summarized in Table 4.1.

4.4 Classes and applications of biomaterials used for dental regeneration

Several classes of biomaterials have been developed for dental tissue regeneration, because of the distinct differences in soft and hard dental tissues, there is no multipurpose biomaterial that can be effectively used for dental pulp regeneration, root perforation repair, periodontal regeneration, gingival regeneration, guided soft-tissue regeneration and bone regeneration.

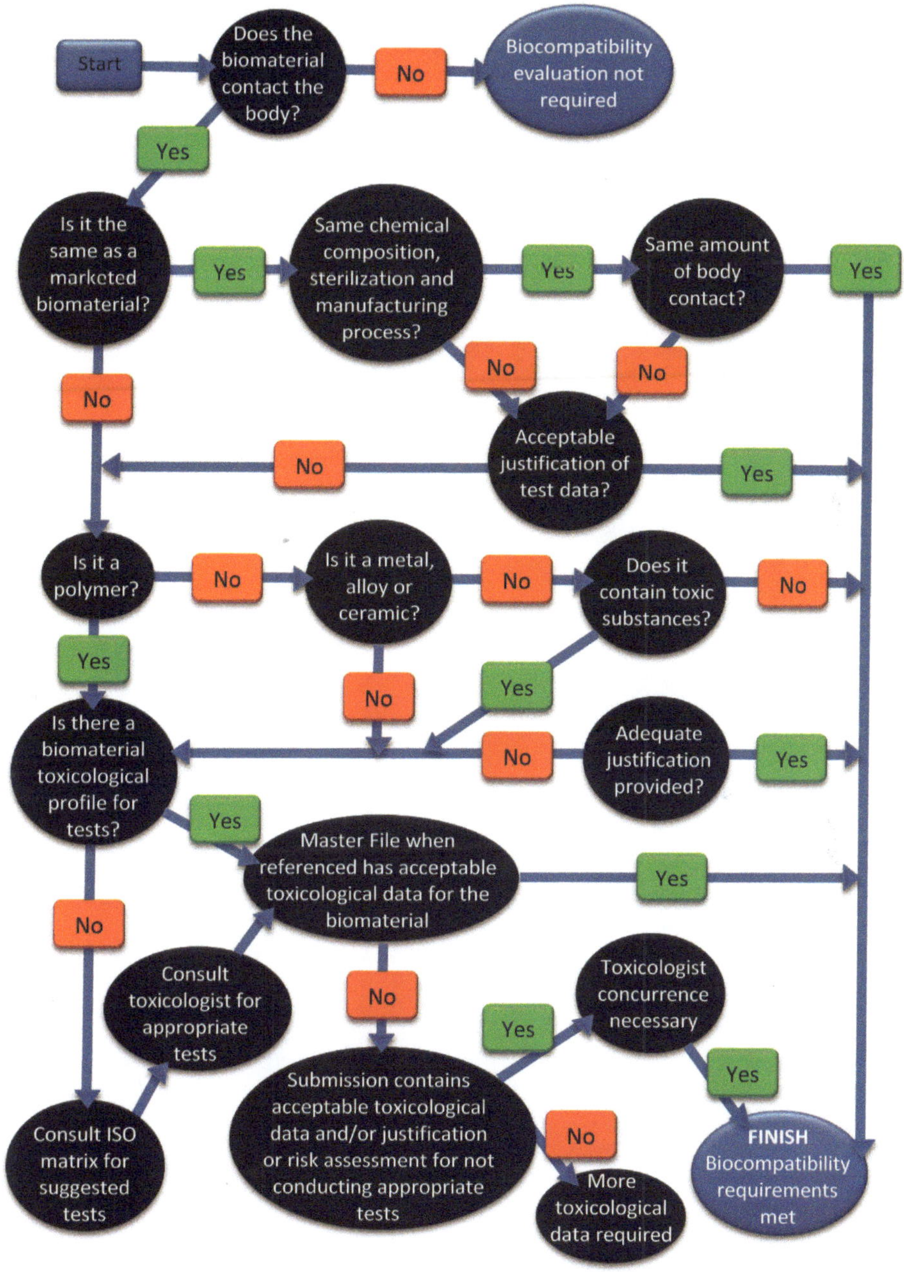
Start
Does the biomaterial contact the body?
No
Biocompatibility evaluation not required
Yes
Is it the same as a marketed biomaterial?
Yes
Same chemical composition, sterilization and manufacturing process?
Yes
Same amount of body contact?
Yes
No
No
No
Acceptable justification of test data?
No
Yes
Is it a polymer?
No
Is it a metal, alloy or ceramic?
No
Does it contain toxic substances?
No
Yes
No
Yes
Is there a biomaterial toxicological profile for tests?
No
Adequate justification provided?
Yes
Yes
Master File when referenced has acceptable toxicological data for the biomaterial
Yes
No
Consult toxicologist for appropriate tests
No
Toxicologist concurrence necessary
Yes
Yes
Submission contains acceptable toxicological data and/or justification or risk assessment for not conducting appropriate tests
Consult ISO matrix for suggested tests
No
More toxicological data required
FINISH
Biocompatibility requirements met

Figure 4.2 Flow chart for guiding the selection of biocompatibility tests for dental repair biomaterials.
Source: Modified from 16: ISO 10993.

Table 4.1 **Biocompatibility testing phases for dental repair biomaterials**

Phase	Type of Test	Example of Test	Tissue source	Test type	Experimental time
1	**Cytotoxicity**	In vitro testing for cytotoxic effect	Permanent cell lines: 3T3, L929	Neutral red exclusion assay	>1 day
	Carcinogenicity and mutagenicity	In vitro testing for carcinogenic or mutagenic effect	Bacterium: *Salmonella typhimurium*	Ames mutagenicity test	<2 days
2	**Irritation, skin sensitization, and systemic toxicity**	Short-term application to non-epithelialized tissue	Small animals: guinea-pigs, rabbits	Topical application	>30 days
		Long-term implantation in subcutaneous tissue in a small animal	Small animals: guinea-pigs, rabbits	Subcutaneous implant	30–70 days
3	**Animal usage experimentation**	Experimentation on animals to mimic the use of the material	Dogs, ferrets, pigs, primates	In situ animal teeth	30–70 days
4	**Clinical experimentation**	Experimentation involving medical procedures on a small group of monitored patients	In situ human teeth	In situ human teeth	More than 1 year

Summarized from ISO 7405, ISO 10993, and the FDA Blue Book Memorandum #G95-1 (25).

4.4.1 Dental pulp and root perforation repair biomaterials

The longest serving biomaterial for dental regeneration is $Ca(OH)_2$, which has become widely used for vital pulp therapy since its introduction to endodontics in 1920 (Hermann, 1920). $Ca(OH)_2$ is a strong alkaline substance, which has a pH of approximately 12.5. $Ca(OH)_2$ has been popular with dentists largely because it is antibacterial, and it can induce pulp healing by mineralization (Foreman and Barnes, 1990). The continued use of $Ca(OH)_2$ as a biomaterial for vital pulp therapy is controversial, although it is inexpensive, it is also highly soluble and has poor physical properties (Niinuma, 1999). $Ca(OH)_2$ is no longer commonly a dentist's first choice of biomaterial for vital pulp procedures, but it is still used extensively for the direct capping of pulp exposures, root perforation repair, and for vital pulp therapies including apexogenesis, Cvek partial pulpotomy, apexification, and regenerative endodontics (Corbella et al., 2014).

Tri-calcium silicate cements such as ProRoot MTA and Biodentine have become the most popular choice for dentists who need a biomaterial for direct pulp capping and for vital pulp therapy procedures (Nowicka et al., 2013). Despite being expensive and slow setting, and sometimes having difficult handling properties, the popularity of MTA has increased rapidly since its development in 1993 (Torabinejad et al., 1993). A good reason why tri-calcium silicate cements have become popular is because they have excellent sealing properties to tooth structure (Torabinejad et al., 1993) which can prevent bacterial microleakage into a vital pulp. Tri-calcium silicate cements are among the dental biomaterials demonstrating biocompatibility (Wälivaara et al., 2012) and this can permit an optimal environment for the healing and regeneration of adjacent tissues. The success of tri-calcium silicate cements in promoting the healing of vital dental tissues may also be because they can stimulate the release of TGF-β1 from dentine (Tomson et al., 2007).

Tri-calcium silicate can be refined into bio-ceramic nanosphere particles to create products such as ESRRM (Damas et al., 2011) and iRoot BP Plus. Similar to MTA, the bio-ceramic tri-calcium silicate is relatively expensive and slow setting, but its main advantages are that it provides good sealing to dentine, and better handling properties since it is supplied in a syringe rather than as a cement powder.

A small number of dentists may be using composite resins, resin-modified glass ionomer, sealers, adhesives, or other types of dental materials for vital pulp therapy and placement in contact with vital tissues. However, those dental materials are potentially much more toxic to tissues and could cause disastrous injury to tissues (Pameijer and Stanley, 1998). Most types of dental materials can leach some potentially toxic chemicals and therefore lack an adequate biocompatibility to be placed in contact with vital tissues. At the present time, the only biomaterials that can be recommended for dental pulp and root perforation repair are $Ca(OH)_2$ and tri-calcium silicate cements.

4.4.2 Periodontal and gingival regeneration biomaterials

The most widely used biomaterial for periodontal and gingival regeneration is an enamel matrix derivative (EMD) called Emdogain, which was first given premarket approval by the FDA in 1996 (Premarket Approval, US Food and Drug Administration, 1996). EMDs contain bioactive proteins called amelogenins from unerupted porcine teeth and these can promote periodontal healing by stimulating systemic inflammatory cells, including macrophages, to release growth factors such as bone morphogenic protein-2 (BMP-2) (Fujishiro et al., 2008). The increased concentrations of BMP-2, amelogenins, and other growth factors around periodontal defects can promote cementogenesis, increase periodontal attachment and can reduce the probing depth of pockets (Sculean et al., 2008). Emdogain is a relatively expensive bioactive material, and since it is now packed in syringes it has good handling properties. Sometimes guided tissue regeneration procedures can be used as an alternative to EMD, but there are none or few other biomaterials that can match the clinical success of EMD.

4.4.3 Guided soft-tissue regeneration biomaterials

Since the 1970s, platelet-rich plasma (PRP) has been prepared by collecting a patient's whole peripheral blood and centrifuging it to create a plasma with a high concentration of platelets (Marx, 2001). Platelets are autologous storage pools of growth factors including cytokines, TGF-ß, and BMP-2, which are locally released to injured tissues (Anitua et al., 2004). The release of growth factors promotes tissue-repair mechanisms such as chemotaxis, cell proliferation, angiogenesis, extracellular matrix deposition, and wound healing (Rozman and Bolta, 2007). Although several in vitro studies, animal studies, and case reports, all generally support the ability of PRP as promoting periodontal tissue regeneration, there have been some clinical studies that have found little benefit to using PRP for periodontal wound healing and bone formation (Choi et al., 2004; Raghoebar et al., 2005). PRP is an autologous, natural, and inexpensive product, but it also requires preparation time, and can increase the time needed to complete each dental procedure by up to 30 minutes.

Resorbable scaffolds and membranes are used for dental guided soft-tissue regeneration, soft-tissue augmentation, wound repair, as well as bone regeneration (Tal et al., 2012). Resorbable scaffolds have been used to dress oral wounds, for closure of graft and extraction sites, and to promote healing. Most of the scaffolds are manufactured from bovine collagen, such as Collacote Wound Dressing Material, although a few other scaffolds for tissue regeneration can be manufactured from synthetic polymers similar to biodegradable surgical sutures (Gotlieb et al., 2008). Collagen membranes are also widely used in periodontal and implant therapy as barriers to prevent epithelial migration and allow cells with regenerative capacity to repopulate the defect area. The placement of scaffolds and membranes into tissue defects can promote the healing and regeneration of soft and hard tissues (Tal et al., 2012) and ultimately they can be completely resorbed by the body.

PRP and EMDs have been advocated as direct pulp capping agents with little apparent success (Orhan et al., 2012). Some other dental materials; $Ca(OH)_2$, tri-calcium silicate cements, composite resins, resin-modified glass ionomer, sealers, and adhesives lack the physical properties needed for soft-tissue regeneration, in addition to lacking adequate biocompatibility. See a summary of the ranking of biocompatibility of dental repair biomaterials in Fig. 4.3.

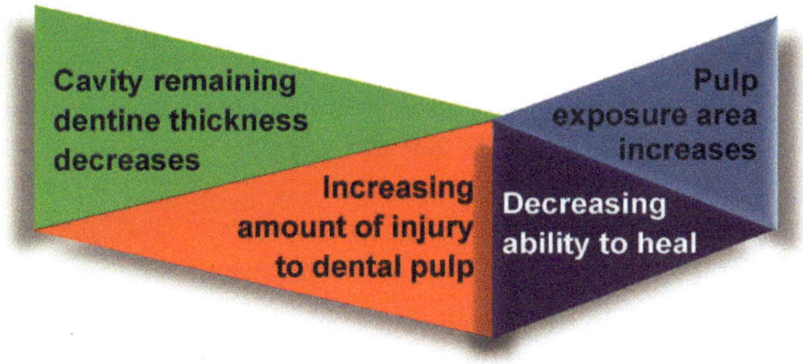

Figure 4.3 Effects of dental biomaterials on dental pulp cell death and repair. The diagram illustrates the relationship observed in restored teeth following cavity preparation and restoration. As the amount of cavity remaining dentine thickness decreases, the amount of pulp injury increases. If the pulp should become exposed, the increasing area of exposure can decrease the ability of the pulp to heal itself.

4.4.4 Bone regeneration biomaterials

Severe bone defects, sometimes called critical-size bone defects, describes a situation where the amount of missing bone is too substantial to be repaired without adding a regeneration biomaterial. Bone regeneration biomaterials are also needed for alveolar ridge preservation to prevent bone loss following tooth extraction, and/or to increase the volume of bone for dental implant placement (Borg and Mealey, 2014). Harvesting a patient's own autologous bone from the iliac crest to autograft into a craniofacial bone defect is a drastic procedure which is no longer necessary or common since the introduction of freeze-dried bone and bone substitute biomaterials demonstrating biocompatibility. Autografting a patient's own bone into a donor site can heal rapidly because of good immunological tolerance. The disadvantages of autografting bone are potential complications arising at the bone harvest site because of surgery and the added cost of surgery.

Demineralized freeze-dried bone allografts (DFDBAs) have excellent de novo bone formation properties and are widely used for periodontal surgery, regenerating alveolar bone to support dental implants, and for reconstruction of bone following trauma, cancer, or a disease. DFDBAs are usually sourced from cadaveric bone donated to a bone bank. The least-common dental allograft bone variants are nondemineralized DFDBA and fresh or fresh-frozen bone. DFDBA has become the most successful biomaterial for bone regeneration because it has good handling properties and is widely regarded as an excellent osteoconductive scaffold. DFDBA could release BMPs which promote bone regeneration, although the amount of BMPs could be in trace amounts and sometimes not be detectable (Li et al., 2000). Overall DFDBA demonstrates biocompatibility at donor sites, and has good immunological tolerance; the main drawback is its high cost.

Bovine bone biomaterials are available for human bone regeneration, such as Bio-Oss which has a similar chemical composition to human bone. The bovine bone biomaterials have earned a reputation for being an effective, safe, reliable, and easy biomaterial to use for regenerating bone in preparation for placing dental implants.

Several synthetic biomaterials are available for bone regeneration; most of the biomaterials contain beta-tricalcium phosphate (β-TCP) and have a similar calcium and phosphate concentration to natural bone. The synthetic bone biomaterials become resorbed by macrophages, phagocytes, and osteoclasts, and through osteogenesis create new bone to fill a bone defect. Sometimes bioactive molecules are added to the graft biomaterials to promote quicker bone regeneration. Some β-TCP biomaterials (GEM 21s, or Augment Bone Graft) contain recombinant human platelet-derived growth factor BB (rhPDGF-BB) which is claimed to be 1000× more concentrated than the growth factors in PRP (Nevins et al., 2005). Another biomaterial (P15 PepGen) coats the β-TCP particles with a synthetic peptide sequence of 15 amino acids (P15) thought to mimic the receptors on osteoblasts to promote osteogenesis (Bhatnagar et al., 1997). Bioactive bone regeneration biomaterials are generally supplied in syringes and are easy to deliver to bone defect sites, but they are often several times more expensive in comparison to biomaterials that do not contain any bioactive molecules. A summary of the main classes of biomaterials for dental regeneration are shown in Table 4.2.

4.5 Applications of dental regeneration biomaterials

4.5.1 Dental biomaterials used for direct pulp capping

Some dental restorative procedures only require a single dental restorative material to accomplish treatment; however, it is uncommon to be able to use a single biomaterial for dental regeneration treatment and also be able to restore the structure of a tooth. When considering the overall biocompatibility of dental biomaterials for regeneration, some consideration must be given to the other chemicals and materials that are used in conjunction with them. Most of the vital tissue regeneration procedures require that the diseased, necrotic, or infected tissue be disinfected prior to placing the regenerative biomaterial. The disinfection of diseased, infected, and necrotic tissues from surgical sites and root canals commonly requires the use of sodium hypochlorite (NaOCl) or chlorhexidine gluconate (CHX). NaOCl is likely to be the most toxic chemical used by most dentists. NaOCl, CHX, and other common disinfectants are cytotoxic to bacteria and human cells. Therefore, NaOCl and CHX must not be allowed to spill or leak into a patient's tissues. To help limit injury to patients if a spill or leak of disinfectant occurs, most dentists will dilute NaOCl from 6% to 3%, or even to 1.5% or lower. The recommended approach to using toxic disinfectants is to use them when needed to remove infected tissues, but to avoid placing them in direct contact with vital tissues. Some potential disinfection agents which are less toxic than NaOCl have been developed, such as natural fruit extracts and electrically activated water, but these are expensive and dentists appear unwilling to switch to using alternative disinfectants.

Dental adhesives, composite resins, sealers, conditioning agents, resin-modified glass ionomers, amalgam, and ZOE are all generally cytotoxic to vital dental tissues and should never be placed in direct contact with vital tissues. If these dental materials come into direct contact with a vital pulp, their cytotoxicity would be expected

Table 4.2 **Classes of biomaterials used for dental tissue regeneration**

Main dental application	Class of dental biomaterial	Chemical composition	Products	Clinical limitations	Clinical advantages
Dental pulp and root perforation repair	**Tri-calcium silicates**	80% Tri-calcium silicate	MTA and Biodentine	Expensive, difficult handling properties, and slow setting	Excellent biocompatibility and sealing to dentine
	Bioceramics	Nanosphere particles of calcium silicate	EndoSequence Root Repair Material	Expensive and slow setting	Excellent biocompatibility, good sealing, easy handling
	Calcium hydroxide materials	100% $Ca(OH)_2$	$Ca(OH)_2$, USB	High solubility, alkalinity	Inexpensive and easy to mix
		25% $Ca(OH)_2$	Life, Dycal	Poor physical properties	Easy handling properties
Periodontal and gingival regeneration	**Porcine growth factor**	Enamel matrix derivative	Emdogain	Expensive	Easy handling properties
Guided soft-tissue regeneration	**Resorbable scaffolds and membranes**	Resorbable collagen or polymers	Collacote, wound dressing	Expensive	Easy handling properties
	Protein-rich plasma	Protein-rich blood plasma or fibrin	Sourced from patient blood	Adds preparation time to collect patients' blood	Natural and inexpensive
Bone regeneration	**Autologous bone**	Patient bone	Patient's own bone	Requires surgical harvesting of bone	Lack of immune rejection reactions
	Demineralized freeze-dried bone allograft	Donor bone	Sourced from donor bone	Expensive	Easy handling properties
	Bone substitute	Bovine bone	Bio-Oss	Expensive	Difficult handling properties
	Bioactive beta-tricalcium phosphate	Beta-tricalcium phosphate with growth factors	GEM 21s and P15 PepGen	Expensive	Easy handling properties

Summarized from the dental literature cited in this chapter.

to cause necrosis of the adjacent pulp tissue, or even a complete eventual necrosis of the dental pulp.

$Ca(OH)_2$ and tri-calcium silicate cements such as MTA and Biodentine demonstrate biocompatibility and are commonly placed in direct contact with a vital dental pulp. $Ca(OH)_2$ and tri-calcium silicate cements are needed to regenerate the pulp tissue as part of direct pulp capping, endodontic revascularization procedures, Cvek partial-pulpotomy apexogenesis, root perforation repair, and periodontal regeneration (Garcia-Godoy and Murray, 2012). A problem with these biomaterials is that they lack the physical properties needed to restore a tooth, and therefore a resin-modified glass ionomer or composite resin must be placed over them to restore a tooth. This means that the biomaterials such as $Ca(OH)_2$ or MTA (demonstrating biocompatibility) must be applied as a liner across an exposed pulp tissue to protect it from the leakage of potentially cytotoxic monomers from the dental material that was used to restore the tooth (Garcia-Godoy and Murray, 2012).

When restoring cavity preparations in teeth, the remaining thickness of dentine separating the floor of the cavity preparation from the dental pulp can act as a protective barrier. A dentine barrier of increased thickness can reduce the amount of potentially cytotoxic chemicals leaching from dental materials into the dental pulp. The increased volume of dental material in a preparation will also increase the quantity of chemicals that can leach from the material. Maintaining the maximal thickness of dentine beneath preparations and minimizing the volume of preparations are key concepts of minimally invasive dentistry, and using them as standard dental procedures could help to minimize pulp injury and adverse events (Murray et al., 2002a). The effects of the remaining dentine thickness and increasing size of pulp exposure in causing increasing pulp injury and a decreased ability to heal is shown in Fig. 4.3.

The other cavity preparation variables which can influence dental pulp cell death and repair the effects of dental biomaterials, include the toxicity of the biomaterials used to restore the preparation, and the absence of coolant during preparation. The other cavity preparation variables such as the heat and vibration induced during the dentine cutting technique, as well as the toxicity of acids and conditioners used to restore the tooth could injure the dental pulp and increase the amount of repair that is needed to maintain its vitality (Murray et al., 2002b). The effects of the dental biomaterials and cavity preparation variables on dental pulp cell death and repair are summarized in Fig. 4.4.

4.5.2 Dental biomaterials used for root canal revascularization and regeneration

Once the pulp of an adult tooth with a closed apex becomes exposed because of trauma or caries decay, its debridement followed by root canal obturation with gutta-percha is an extremely successful procedure (Salehrabi and Rotstein, 2004). In the immature traumatized teeth of children with a necrotic pulp, an apexification procedure can help avoid the risk of pain and necrotic pulp complications from developing (Guzeler et al., 2010). The problem with apexification is that it does not regenerate tooth structure, so an immature tooth can have weak dentine walls which are prone to

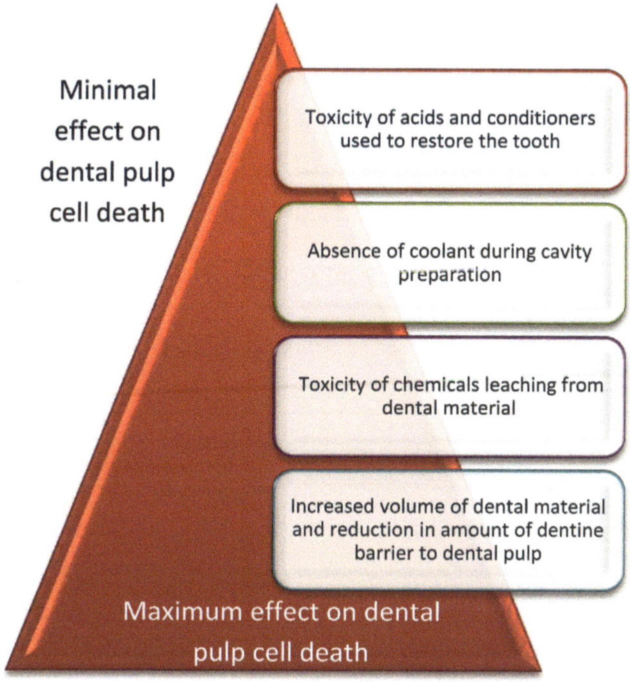

Figure 4.4 Effects of dental biomaterials and interactions with other cavity preparation variables on dental pulp cell death. The relationship is that as the remaining dentine thickness decrease, the amount of dentine barrier is reduced and this can allow an increase in the leaching of chemicals into the pulp. The greater the amount of dental material in the restoration; the greater quantity of chemicals that can leach out. The toxicity of the chemicals able to leach from a dental material can also injure the dental pulp by causing cell death. Cutting preparations without coolant can cause thermal injury to the dental pulp. The toxicity of acids and conditioners used in adhesives to bond restorative materials can also cause injury to the pulp.

fracture. An alternative dental procedure called root canal revascularization or regeneration can be used to replace the necrotic pulp with a replacement tissue which can promote dentin wall thickening and root development, thus strengthening the structure of the tooth to help resist fracture (Garcia-Godoy and Murray, 2012). Root canal revascularization or regeneration requires the disinfection of the root canal by rinsing it with NaOCl. Further disinfection of the root canal can be accomplished by obturating it with an antibiotic paste for 4 weeks or $Ca(OH)_2$ in some cases, or by using endodontic files and instruments to remove the necrotic tissues. After the root canal is cleaned and disinfected, a file is placed beyond the apex to cause bleeding from the periapical tissues into the root canal. The blood will be allowed to form a blood clot inside the root canal to serve as a scaffold for tissue regeneration. Sometimes a collagen scaffold will be placed inside the blood clot to help promote tissue regeneration. Above the blood clot in the coronal access, MTA can be placed as thin layer; its purpose is to allow tissue regeneration within the root canal. The MTA is also used to

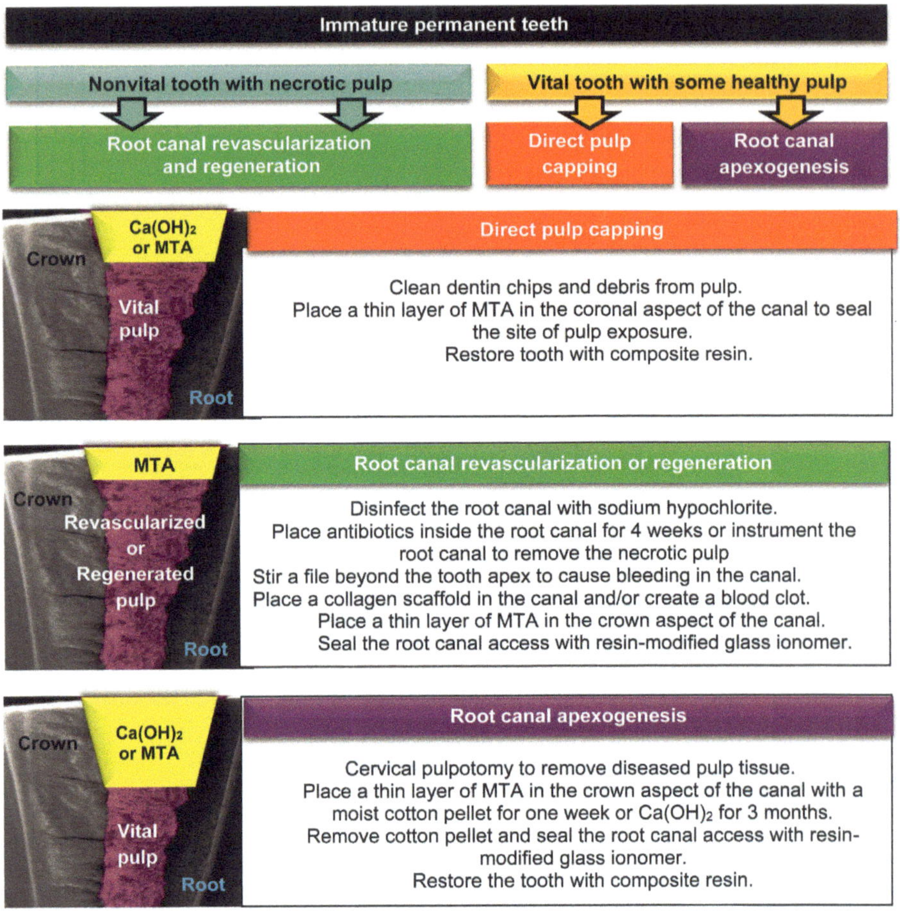

Figure 4.5 Applications of dental pulp regeneration biomaterials for the direct pulp capping, root canal revascularization/regeneration, or apexogenesis for immature permanent teeth.

seal the access to the root canal and prevent microleakage. Above the MTA, the access can be restored with a glass ionomer or sometimes a composite resin. The steps for using dental biomaterials for root canal revascularization and regeneration are shown in Fig. 4.5.

4.5.3 Dental biomaterials used for root canal apexogenesis

Sometimes an immature tooth with a vital pulp can become injured by trauma, with a fracture through the crown above the cemento-enamel junction. In these teeth, some dentists will perform a Cvek pulpotomy to remove 2 mm of dental pulp (Cvek, 1978), other dentists will place $Ca(OH)_2$ in contact with the exposed dental pulp to promote its calcification (Aggarwal et al., 2012). The $Ca(OH)_2$ has to be replaced every 3 months and will often be replaced three times before the tooth is given a final restoration (Aggarwal et al., 2012). Some dentists will not perform a Cvek pulpotomy or use $Ca(OH)_2$ (Cvek, 1978); instead they will place MTA in contact with the pulp tissue with a moist cotton pellet for 3 days or longer, and then remove the cotton pellet and restore the teeth (Khalilak et al., 2012). The goal of an apexogenesis protocol is to promote the continued root development, which some researchers call maturogenesis (Weisleder and Benitez, 2003). The outcome of the apexogenesis procedure is reliable if the majority of the pulp tissue in the roots of teeth are healthy and vital (Chueh and Huang, 2006). The steps for using dental biomaterials for apexogenesis are shown in Fig. 4.5.

4.6 Biocompatibility of dental regeneration materials

Most dentists have concerns about the potential toxic effects of handling restorative dental biomaterials; 24% of dentists believe that dental materials will cause themselves no health effects, 39% of dentists believe that dental materials can poison themselves temporarily, and 37% of dentists believe that dental materials could poison themselves permanently (unpublished data). In addition, most dentists have concerns about the potential toxic effects of restorative dental biomaterials on the health of their patients: 45% believe that dental materials will have no health effects on their dental patients, 34% believe that dental materials can poison patients temporarily, and 21% believe that dental materials can poison patients permanently (unpublished data). Given all the concerns that dentists have about protecting their own health and the health of their patients, it is important to know which dental materials demonstrate biocompatibility.

The biocompatibility of dental repair biomaterials can vary greatly with the most toxic generally being ZOE. ZOE is widely regarded to be the acceptable limit for how toxic a dental material can be, thus ZOE also sets the standard for biocompatibility: any dental materials that are more toxic than ZOE do not have an acceptable biocompatibility, and materials that are less toxic than ZOE have an acceptable toxicity (ISO 7405, 2008). Endodontic sealers, adhesives, etching, and conditioning agents are often less toxic than ZOE, but can still be toxic to vital pulp tissues and cause disastrous pulp necrosis (Pameijer and Stanley, 1998). Endodontic sealers, adhesives, etching, and conditioning agents should never be placed in direct contact with vital tissues because of their relatively high toxicity, in order to prevent avoidable adverse reactions. Amalgam, and glass ionomers or resin-glass ionomers are not as toxic as the previous list of dental materials, but they still lack an adequate biocompatiblility to be placed in direct contact with the dental pulp or other vital tissues.

The best and least toxic dental biomaterials formulated for vital pulp therapy are tri-calcium silicate cements; including MTA and related bio-ceramic biomaterials, such as ESRRM. During the past decade, MTA has replaced $Ca(OH)_2$ as the first choice of biomaterial for placing in contact with a vital pulp (Garcia-Godoy and Murray, 2012). MTA has a low toxicity and good sealing properties to prevent microleakage (Torabinejad et al., 1993; Khalilak et al., 2012). MTA can also stimulate the release of growth factors, which promotes the healing and repair of vital pulp tissues (Tomson et al., 2007). Other biomaterials, such as Emdogain for periodontal regeneration, and PepGen P15 for bone augmentation contain active growth factors to promote tissue regeneration (Emam et al., 2011). Successful dental repair materials must lack toxicity, demonstrate biocompatibility, not induce inflammation sensitivity or pain, be physically stable and seal to prevent bacterial microleakage, and promote tissue repair by creating an environment where growth factors can induce stem cells and local cells to heal injured tissues. The in vitro culture of periodontal stem cells was used as a screening method (ISO 7405) to test the cytotoxicity of biomaterials. The least to the most cytotoxic biomaterials were: MTA (76%), amalgam (42%), composite (35%), glass ionomer (28%), $Ca(OH)_2$ (16%) and ZOE (11%) (unpublished data) as seen in Fig. 4.6.

What is interesting about MTA is that although it is widely regarded to be the most suitable biomaterial for vital pulp therapy (Garcia-Godoy and Murray, 2012) and vital periodontal therapy, it still does not allow 100% survival of the cells it is placed into contact with. It seems unrealistic to expect any dental biomaterial when used following a vital tissue injury to be able to maintain 100% survival of injured cells, but MTA appears to do this best, particularly when compared with other biomaterials. The 16% survival rate of periodontal cells in response to $Ca(OH)_2$ may be considered to be surprising, considering that it is still often used for vital pulp therapy. The answer is that $Ca(OH)_2$ demonstrates a degree of biocompatibility, but it is also highly alkaline and causes the necrosis of adjacent tissues, hence the low cell survival seen in Fig. 4.6. Clearly, using any other dental biomaterial (amalgam, composite resin, glass ionomer, $Ca(OH)_2$, or ZOE) for root perforation repair, or vital pulp therapy instead of MTA will likely result in more cell death within the vital periodontal tissue or vital pulp tissue. Hence, at this present time, most dentists are using

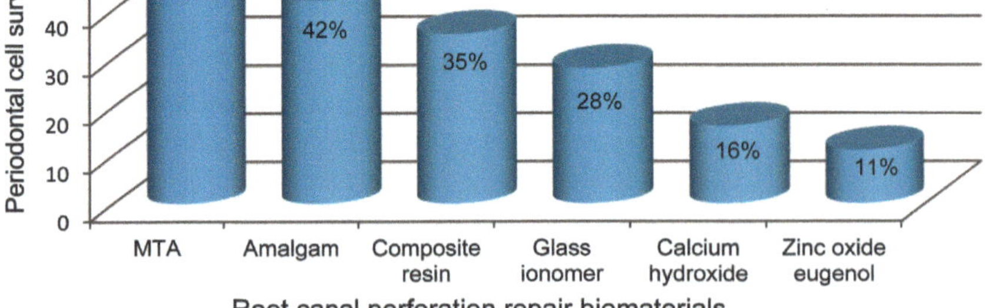

Figure 4.6 Toxicity of root canal perforation biomaterials according to periodontal cell survival.

MTA as the biomaterial of choice to help prevent vital dental treatment failure and the risks of complications.

Sometimes MTA is not adequate for vital dental tissue repair, because the regeneration of missing or diseased tissues is necessary to accomplish healing. An increasing skill is to use scaffolds and membranes as part of guided tissue regeneration treatments. Generally, the scaffolds for tissue regeneration can be divided into two types: spongy scaffolds which can be molded into dental tissue defects, and liquid scaffolds which can be injected into tissue defects. The most common types of spongy biodegradable scaffolds are plastic polymers such as OPLA (Open-cell, PolyLactic Acid) (Di Felice et al., 2009), or calcium phosphate, which is normally an ideal scaffold for bone regeneration or sometimes dental pulp regeneration (AbdulQader et al., 2015), or bovine collagen (Fawzy El-Sayed et al., 2012) which mimics the human natural collagen scaffold. Some common liquid scaffolds include demineralized bone matrix (Rhee et al., 2011), PepGen P15 (Butz et al., 2011), and an alginate hydrogel (Moshaverinia et al., 2012). An unpublished histologic comparison of dental pulp cell and periodontal cell vitality (by a former NSU resident, Dr Glorimar Llavona) within the spongy and liquid scaffolds, suggests that the spongy scaffolds are more effective in promoting cell vitality, as seen in Fig. 4.7.

In addition to the use of spongy and liquid scaffolds, there is also the collection of a patient's own peripheral blood to create PRP scaffolds (Bezgin et al., 2015). The PRP scaffolds have a mixed record of success and can add 30 minutes of waiting time to prepare it, hence the preference of most dentists for using spongy scaffolds when vital tissue regeneration is required.

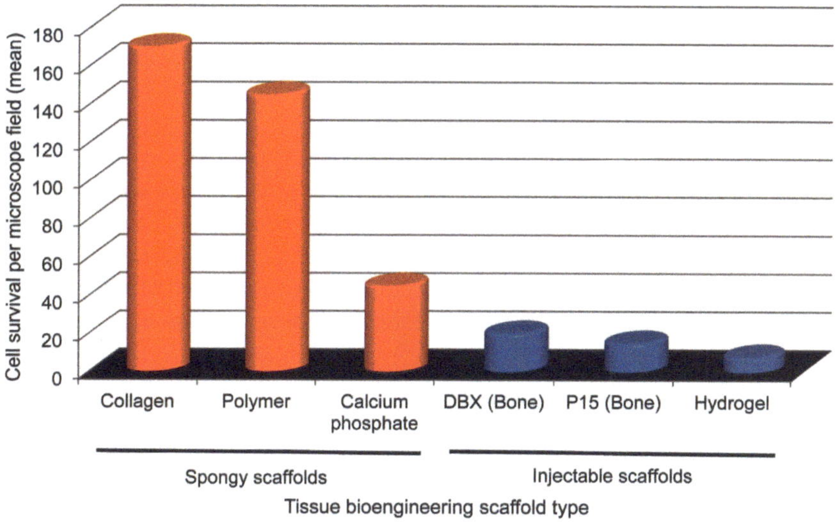

Figure 4.7 Cell vitality within spongy and injectable scaffolds.

4.7 Challenges for developing improved dental regeneration materials

Fortunately, dentists and patients are giving their full attention to the safety of dental biomaterials, through the amalgam controversy (Mackey et al., 2014), and the media attention of potential severe allergic reactions (Liu, 2014). For most of the history of modern dentistry, $Ca(OH)_2$ has been the most widely used dental biomaterial for vital pulp therapy (Foreman and Barnes, 1990). However, as seen in this chapter, it does not demonstrate optimal biocompatibility to cells or vital tissues because its high alkalinity causes localized tissue necrosis (Turner et al., 1987). The demise of $Ca(OH)_2$ as the biomaterial for vital pulp therapy began in 1995, with the development of tri-calcium silicate cements such as MTA (Torabinejad et al., 1995). Over the years, there have been polymerizers added to MTA to speed up its long setting time and to improve its handling properties (Chung et al., 2015). The trend of modifying MTA to improve its suitability for dental regeneration is likely to continue long into the future.

The reason for the success of tri-calcium silicate cements for vital pulp therapy is not just their biocompatibility, but also their ability stimulate the release of growth factors in adjacent tissues and the growth factors found in dentine (Tomson et al., 2007), such as TGF-β1 which can promote tissue healing and regeneration (Dobie et al., 2002). A promising area of research is the development of biomaterials, membranes, and scaffolds which release bioactive compounds such as Emdogain (Abbas et al., 2003) to promote periodontal regeneration and P-15 to promote bone regeneration (Emam et al., 2011). A major limitation of bioactive compounds is their high price which limits their widespread use in dental treatments. The relatively high price of bioactive compounds is unlikely to change in the near future, hence the search among researchers for low-cost biomaterials demonstrating biocompatibility. This helps to explain the novel dental biomaterials that are being developed from cheap raw materials such as chitosan (Hamilton et al., 2014).

Many researchers believe the transformational wave of nanotechnology will drastically alter the chemical, physical, optical, wear, antibacterial, and polymerization properties of composite dental biomaterials (Mohamed Hamouda, 2012). Nanoparticles are clusters of atoms in the size range of 1–100 nm. Most nanomaterials are being developed from metals to create antibacterial materials that can prevent the growth of bacteria (Grumezescu and Chifiriuc, 2014). A problem with nanomaterials is that regulators are concerned about their safety, because of the potential of the nanoparticles to disperse freely and cause harmful or benign reactions (Tyner et al., 2015). Only once nanomaterials are proven to be safe, and effective can dentists and patients benefit from the exciting dental biomaterial developments that nanotechnology will make possible.

4.8 Conclusions

Dentists have an extensive array of materials at their disposal, but only a few of those biomaterials have a lack of toxicity and biocompatibility to be used for vital pulp therapies, perforation repair, and for dental regeneration. Historically, dentists have been cautious in selecting biomaterials for vital pulp therapy and tissue repair, which highlights the continuing need for dentists to receive training in the use of new biomaterials for dental tissue regeneration.

During the history of dentistry, the introduction of new materials has taken a long time to become widely accepted. Even today, almost no one agrees on the safety of amalgam, and it has been controversial for over a century. Only within the past two decades have scaffolds, membranes, and tri-calcium silicate cements become available to allow dentists to deliver regenerative dental treatments to patients. Bioactive materials such as PepGen P-15 and Emdogain will always have some demand in dental tissue repair, but their use is limited by their relatively high cost. The introduction of nanotechnology into dental materials has already began and its spread to all biomaterials is inevitable, if the safety concerns can be addressed. Nanotechnology has the potential to create hard-wearing, long-lasting biomaterials which can resist infection. Biomaterials engineered with nanotechnology could help dentists to deliver even more successful dental regeneration treatments to their future patients.

References

Abbas, F., Wennström, J., Van der Weijden, F., Schneiders, T., Van der Velden, U., 2003. Surgical treatment of gingival recessions using emdogain gel: clinical procedure and case reports. Int. J. Periodontics Restorative Dent. 23, 607–613.

AbdulQader, S.T., Kannan, T.P., Rahman, I.A., Ismail, H., Mahmood, Z., 2015. Effect of different calcium phosphate scaffold ratios on odontogenic differentiation of human dental pulp cells. Mater. Sci. Eng. C Mater. Biol. Appl. 49, 225–233.

Aggarwal, V., Miglani, S., Singla, M., 2012. Conventional apexification and revascularization induced maturogenesis of two non-vital, immature teeth in same patient: 24 months follow up of a case. J. Conserv. Dent. 15, 68–72.

Anitua, E., Andia, I., Ardanza, B., Nurden, P., Nurden, A.T., 2004. Autologous platelets as a source of proteins for healing and tissue regeneration. Thromb. Haemost. 91, 4–15.

Bezgin, T., Yilmaz, A.D., Celik, B.N., Kolsuz, M.E., Sonmez, H., 2015. Efficacy of platelet-rich plasma as a scaffold in regenerative endodontic treatment. J. Endod. 41, 36–44.

Bhatnagar, R.S., Qian, J.J., Gough, C.A., 1997. The role in cell-binding of a a-bend within the triple helical region in collagen b1(I) chain: structural and biological evidence for conformational tautomerism on fiber surface. J. Biomol. Struct. Dyn. 14, 547–560.

Borg, T.D., Mealey, B.L., 2014. Histologic healing following tooth extraction with ridge preservation using mineralized freeze dried bone allograft alone versus a combined mineralized-demineralized freeze dried bone allograft. A randomized controlled clinical trial. J. Periodontol. 21, 1–13.

Butz, F., Bächle, M., Ofer, M., Marquardt, K., Kohal, R.J., 2011. Sinus augmentation with bovine hydroxyapatite/synthetic peptide in a sodium hyaluronate carrier (PepGen P-15 Putty): a clinical investigation of different healing times. Int. J. Oral Maxillofac. Implants 26, 1317–1323.

Choi, B.H., Im, C.J., Huh, J.Y., Suh, J.J., Lee, S.H., 2004. Effect of platelet-rich plasma on bone regeneration in autogenous bone graft. Int. J. Oral Maxillofac. Surg. 33, 56–59.

Chueh, L.H., Huang, G.T., 2006. Immature teeth with periradicular periodontitis or abscess undergoing apexogenesis: a paradigm shift. J. Endod. 32, 1205–1213.

Chung, C.J., Kim, E., Song, M., Park, J.W., Shin, S.J., 2015. Effects of two fast-setting calcium-silicate cements on cell viability and angiogenic factor release in human pulp-derived cells. Odontology 104 (2), 143–151.
Corbella, S., Ferrara, G., El Kabbaney, A., Taschieri, S., 2014. Apexification, apexogenesis and regenerative endodontic procedures: a review of the literature. Minerva. Stomatol. 63, 375–389.
Cox, C.F., Keall, C.L., Keall, H.J., Ostro, E., Bergenholtz, G., 1987. Biocompatibility of surface-sealed dental materials against exposed pulps. J. Prosthet. Dent. 57, 1–8.
Cvek, M., 1978. A clinical report on partial pulpotomy and capping with calcium hydroxide in permanent incisors with complicated crown fracture. J. Endod. 4, 232–237.
Damas, B.A., Wheater, M.A., Bringas, J.S., Hoen, M.M., 2011. Cytotoxicity comparison of mineral trioxide aggregates and EndoSequence bioceramic root repair materials. J. Endod. 37, 372–375.
Di Felice, V., Ardizzone, N.M., De Luca, A., Marcianò, V., Marino Gammazza, A., Macaluso, F., et al., 2009. OPLA scaffold, collagen I, and horse serum induce an higher degree of myogenic differentiation of adult rat cardiac stem cells. J. Cell Physiol. 221, 729–739.
Dobie, K., Smith, G., Sloan, A.J., Smith, A.J., 2002. Effects of alginate hydrogels and TGF-beta 1 on human dental pulp repair in vitro. Connect Tissue Res. 43, 387–390.
Emam, H., Beheiri, G., Elsalanty, M., Sharawy, M., 2011. Microcomputed tomographic and histologic analysis of anorganic bone matrix coupled with cell-binding peptide suspended in sodium hyaluronate carrier after sinus augmentation: a clinical study. Int. J. Oral Maxillofac. Implants 26, 561–570.
Fawzy El-Sayed, K.M., Paris, S., Becker, S.T., Neuschl, M., De Buhr, W., Sälzer, S., et al., 2012. Periodontal regeneration employing gingival margin-derived stem/progenitor cells: an animal study. J. Clin. Periodontol. 39, 861–870.
Foreman, P.C., Barnes, I.E., 1990. Review of calcium hydroxide. Int. Endod. J. 23, 283–297.
Fujishiro, N., Anan, H., Hamachi, T., Maeda, K., 2008. The role of macrophages in the periodontal regeneration using Emdogain gel. J. Period. Res. 43, 143–155.
Garcia-Godoy, F., Murray, P.E., 2012. Recommendations for using regenerative endodontic procedures in permanent immature traumatized teeth. Dent. Traumatol. 28, 33–41.
Geurtsen, W., 2000. Biocompatibility of resin-modified filling materials. Crit. Rev. Oral Biol. Med. 11, 333–355.
Gotlieb, E.L., Murray, P.E., Namerow, K.N., Kuttler, S., Garcia-Godoy, F., 2008. An ultrastructural investigation of tissue-engineered pulp constructs implanted within endodontically treated teeth. J. Am. Dent. Assoc. 139, 457–465.
Grumezescu, A.M., Chifiriuc, C.M., 2014. Prevention of microbial biofilms—the contribution of micro and nanostructured materials. Curr. Med. Chem. 21, 3311.
Guzeler, I., Uysal, S., Cehreli, Z.C., 2010. Management of trauma-induced inflammatory root resorption using mineral trioxide aggregate obturation: two-year follow up. Dent. Traumatol. 26, 501–504.
Hamilton, M.F., Otte, A.D., Gregory, R.L., Pinal, R., Ferreira-Zandoná, A., Bottino, M.C., 2014. Physicomechanical and antibacterial properties of experimental resin-based dental sealants modified with nylon-6 and chitosan nanofibers. J. Biomed. Mater. Res. B Appl. Biomater. 103 (8), 1560–1568.
Hensten-Pettersen, A., Helgeland, K., 1977. Evaluation of biologic effects of dental materials using four different cell culture techniques. Scand. J. Dent. Res. 85, 291–296.
Hermann, B.W., 1920. Calciumhydroxyd Als Mittel Zum Behandein und Fullen Von Zahnwurzelkanalen (Dissertation). Wurzburg, Germany.
ISO 7405, 2008. Dentistry—Evaluation of Biocompatibility of Medical Devices Used in Dentistry. International Organization for Standization, Geneva.

ISO 10993, 2010. Biological Evaluation of Medical Devices. International Standards Organization, Geneva.

Khalilak, Z., Vali, T., Danesh, F., Vatanpour, M., 2012. The effect of one-step or two-step MTA plug and tooth apical width on coronal leakage in open apex teeth. Iran Endod. J. 7, 10–14.

Kostoryz, E.L., Eick, J.D., Glaros, A.G., Judy, B.M., Welshons, W.V., Burmaster, S., et al., 2003. Biocompatibility of hydroxylated metabolites of BISGMA and BFDGE. J. Dent. Res. 82, 367–371.

Li, H., Pujic, Z., Xiao, Y., Bartold, P.M., 2000. Identification of bone morphogenetic proteins 2 and 4 in commercial demineralized freeze-dried bone allograft preparations: pilot study. Clin. Implant Dent. Relat. Res. 2, 110–117.

Liu, K., 2014. [Emergency treatment of severe allergic reactions in dental clinic] Article in Chinese. Zhonghua Kou Qiang Yi Xue Za Zhi 49, 693–697.

Mackey, T.K., Contreras, J.T., Liang, B.A., 2014. The minamata convention on Mercury: attempting to address the global controversy of dental amalgam use and mercury waste disposal. Sci. Total Environ. 472, 125–129.

Marx, R.E., 2001. Platelet-rich plasma (PRP): what is PRP and what is not PRP? Implant Dent. 10, 225–228.

Mjor, I.A., 1992. Problems and benefits associated with restorative materials: side-effects and long-term cost. Adv. Dent. Res. 6, 7–16.

Mohamed Hamouda, I., 2012. Current perspectives of nanoparticles in medical and dental biomaterials. J. Biomed. Res. 26, 143–151.

Moshaverinia, A., Chen, C., Akiyama, K., Ansari, S., Xu, X., Chee, W.W., et al., 2012. Alginate hydrogel as a promising scaffold for dental-derived stem cells: an in vitro study. J. Mater. Sci. Mater. Med. 23, 3041–3051.

Müller, J., Bruckner, G., Kraft, E., Hörz, W., 1990. Reaction of cultured pulp cells to eight different cements based on glass ionomers. Dent. Mater. 6, 172–177.

Murray, P.E., Hafez, A.A., Smith, A.J., Cox, C.F., 2002a. Hierarchy of pulp capping and repair activities responsible for dentin bridge formation. Am. J. Dent. 15, 236–243.

Murray, P.E., Windsor, L.J., Smyth, T.W., Hafez, A.A., Cox, C.F., 2002b. Analysis of pulpal reactions to restorative procedures, materials, pulp capping, and future therapies. Crit. Rev. Oral Biol. Med. 13, 509–520.

Murray, P.E., Hafez, A.A., Smith, A.J., Cox, C.F., 2003. Identification of hierarchical factors to guide clinical decision making for successful long-term pulp capping. Quintessence Int. 34, 61–70.

Murray, P.E., García-Godoy, C., García-Godoy, F., 2007. How is the biocompatibility of dental biomaterials evaluated? Med. Oral Patol Oral Cir. Bucal. 12, E258–E266.

Neupert, G., Welker, D., 1980. Toxicity evaluation of water soluble substances of dental materials by means of cell population in vitro. Arch. Toxicol. Suppl. 4, 410–412.

Nevins, M., Giannobile, W.V., McGuire, M.K., Kao, R.T., Mellonig, J.T., Hinrichs, J.E., et al., 2005. Platelet derived growth factor (rhPDGF-BB) stimulates bone fill and rate of attachment level gain. Results of a large, multicenter randomized controlled trial. J. Periodontol. 76, 2205–2215.

Niinuma, A., 1999. Newly developed resinous direct pulp capping agent containing calcium hydroxide (MTYA1-Ca). Int. Endod. J. 32, 475–483.

Nowicka, A., Lipski, M., Parafiniuk, M., Sporniak-Tutak, K., Lichota, D., Kosierkiewicz, A., et al., 2013. Response of human dental pulp capped with biodentine and mineral trioxide aggregate. J. Endod. 39, 743–747.

Orhan, E.O., Maden, M., Senguüven, B., 2012. Odontoblast-like cell numbers and reparative dentine thickness after direct pulp capping with platelet-rich plasma and enamel matrix derivative: a histomorphometric evaluation. Int. Endod. J. 45, 317–325.

Pameijer, C.H., Stanley, H.R., 1998. The disastrous effects of the "total etch" technique in vital pulp capping in primates. Am. J. Dent. (11 Spec No), S45–S54.
Raghoebar, G.M., Schortinghuis, J., Liem, R.S., Ruben, J.L., van der Wal, J.E., Vissink, A., 2005. Does platelet-rich plasma promote remodeling of autologous bone grafts used for augmentation of the maxillary sinus floor? Clin. Oral Implants Res. 16, 349–356.
Rhee, S.C., Ji, Y.H., Gharibjanian, N.A., Dhong, E.S., Park, S.H., Yoon, E.S., 2011. In vivo evaluation of mixtures of uncultured freshly isolated adipose-derived stem cells and demineralized bone matrix for bone regeneration in a rat critically sized calvarial defect model. Stem Cells Dev. 20, 233–242.
Ribeiro, D.A., Sugui, M.M., Matsumoto, M.A., Duarte, M.A., Marques, M.E., Salvadori, D.M., 2006. Genotoxicity and cytotoxicity of mineral trioxide aggregate and regular and white Portland cements on Chinese hamster ovary (CHO) cells in vitro. Oral Surg. Oral Med. Oral Pathol. Oral Radiol. Endod. 101, 258–261.
Rozman, P., Bolta, Z., 2007. Use of platelet growth factors in treating wounds and soft-tissue injuries. Acta Dermatovenerol Alp Pannonica Adriat. 16, 156–165.
Salehrabi, R., Rotstein, I., 2004. Endodontic treatment outcomes in a large patient population in the USA: an epidemiological study. J. Endod. 30, 846–850.
Sculean, A., Windisch, P., Szendröi-Kiss, D., Horváth, A., Rosta, P., Becker, J., et al., 2008. Clinical and histologic evaluation of an enamel matrix derivative combined with a biphasic calcium phosphate for the treatment of human intrabony periodontal defects. J. Periodontol. 79, 1991–1999.
Tal, H., Moses, O., Kozlovsky, A., Nemcovsky, C., 2012. Bioresorbable collagen membranes for guided bone regeneration. In: Tal, H. (Ed.), Bone Regeneration. InTech, Rijeka, pp. 111–138.
Tomson, P.L., Grover, L.M., Lumley, P.J., Sloan, A.J., Smith, A.J., Cooper, P.R., 2007. Dissolution of bio-active dentine matrix components by mineral trioxide aggregate. J. Dent. 35, 636–642.
Torabinejad, M., Hong, C.U., McDonald, F., Pitt-Ford, T.R., 1995. Physical and chemical properties of a new root-end filling material. J. Endod. 21, 349–353.
Torabinejad, M., Watson, T.F., Pitt-Ford, T.R., 1993. Sealing ability of mineral trioxide aggregate when used as a root end filling material. J. Endod. 19, 591–595.
Turner, C., Courts, F.J., Stanley, H.R., 1987. A histological comparison of direct pulp capping agents in primary canines. ASDC J. Dent. Child. 54, 423–428.
Tyner, K.M., Zou, P., Yang, X., Zhang, H., Cruz, C.N., Lee, S.L., 2015. Product quality for nanomaterials: current U.S. experience and perspective. Wiley Interdiscip Rev. Nanomed. Nanobiotechnol. 7 (5), 640–654.
US Food and Drug Administration Premarket Approval (PMA), 1996. Biora Emdogain. Washington, DC.
Wälivaara, D.Å., Abrahamsson, P., Isaksson, S., Salata, L.A., Sennerby, L., Dahlin, C., 2012. Periapical tissue response after use of intermediate restorative material, gutta-percha, reinforced zinc oxide cement, and mineral trioxide aggregate as retrograde root-end filling materials: a histologic study in dogs. J. Oral Maxillofac. Surg. 70, 2041–2047.
Weisleder, R., Benitez, C.R., 2003. Maturogenesis: is it a new concept? J. Endod. 29, 776–778.
Witherspoon, D.E., 2008. Vital pulp therapy with new materials: new directions and treatment perspectives–permanent teeth. Pediatr. Dent. 30, 220–224.

Biocompatibility and functionality of dental restorative materials

5

A. Zabrovsky, N. Beyth*, Y. Pietrokovski, G. Ben-Gal and Y. Houri-Haddad*
The Hebrew University-Hadassah School of Dental Medicine, Jerusalem, Israel

Abstract

Dental restorative materials are required to fulfill basic prerequisites including similarity to tooth structures in their mechanical, physical, and esthetic properties. Although dental restorative materials differ significantly in their characteristics, they are all, once placed as restorations, subjected to the harsh conditions of the oral cavity. After placement, dental restorative materials are in constant interaction with the surrounding tissues. Although dental restorative materials are fabricated to be as durable and inert as possible, restorations may deteriorate, degrade or fail, and during these processes, constituents of these materials may be released into the oral cavity. Not only are these materials expected to maintain their integrity in such harsh conditions, but also to preserve these features during function for prolonged periods. As most restorative materials have a long lifespan, their functionality may alter their basic properties, including those related to biocompatibility. Restorative materials in function need to endure chewing forces, aqueous conditions, numerous microorganisms, fluctuations in pH, food products, temperature swings, and active enzymes. This chapter discusses the general functionality principles of the different material groups in relation to their biocompatibility.

Chapter Outline

*The authors have equally contributed to this chapter.

Biocompatibility of Dental Biomaterials. DOI: http://dx.doi.org/10.1016/B978-0-08-100884-3.00005-9

5.1 Introduction

Dental restorative materials are required to fulfill basic prerequisites including similarity to tooth structures in their mechanical, physical, and esthetic properties. Although dental restorative materials differ significantly in their characteristics, they are all, once placed as restorations, subjected to the harsh conditions of the oral cavity. After placement, dental restorative materials are in constant interaction with the surrounding tissues. Although dental restorative materials are fabricated to be as durable and inert as possible, restorations may deteriorate, degrade or fail, and during these processes, constituents of these materials may be released into the oral cavity. Not only are these materials expected to maintain their integrity in such harsh conditions, but also to preserve these features during function for prolonged periods. As most restorative materials have a long lifespan, their functionality may alter their basic properties, including those related to biocompatibility. Restorative materials in function need to endure chewing forces, aqueous conditions, numerous microorganisms, fluctuations in pH, food products, temperature swings, and active enzymes. This chapter discusses the general functionality principles of the different material groups in relation to their biocompatibility.

5.2 Mastication

While functioning, restorative materials undergo recurrent loading and unloading, i.e., repeated loading. The material itself is exposed to mechanical loading and its surface is affected by the extent and direction of the loading, both of which contribute to the stress and strain within the material as well as surface wear. In the course of mastication, restorative materials are constantly exposed to mechanical and thermal cycles and, under such challenges, these undergo fatigue and may release various components from the bulk material.

The site of the restoration constitutes an important consideration in the total wear process during function. Two-body wear can be seen at the buccal and lingual tooth sites where restorations are exposed to tooth brushing abrasion or at the contact point sites between the teeth. Three-body wear can be found at the occlusal areas during mastication.

During the mastication process, teeth and restoration surfaces contact and interact, resulting in continuous substance loss and wear. Biocompatibility may be affected by the interaction conditions, which change according to the physical and mechanical challenges, as well as to environmental factors. Environmental conditions within the mouth are diverse and are modified by saliva, food type, microorganisms, pH, enzymes, and temperature.

5.3 Saliva

Saliva plays provides a fluid layer between the sliding surfaces that reduce the friction encountered during mastication (Mandel, 1987). Human saliva also serves as a buffer, ion reservoir, and aids digestion. Saliva exhibits lubricating properties attributed to its charged, extended macromolecules, including glycoproteins and high-molecular-weight proteins (Hatton et al., 1985). The film produced by these salivary constituents coats the restoration material and generates surface endurance against substances sliding on it, thus reducing biocompatibility alterations because of wear (Aguirre et al., 1989).

Saliva also plays a role as a protective barrier against acidic activity by acting as a buffer (Mandel, 1987). However, during function saliva can change from mildly alkaline to strongly acidic. During prolonged exposure to acid, some of the constituents of saliva and other solvents, such as acids and organic fluids, can cause chemical degradation of dental restorations by penetrating it and reacting with it chemically. Nonetheless, it is considered that salivary and microbial enzymes have a greater effect on the biocompatibility of restorative materials than water and chemicals present in the oral environment.

5.4 Microorganisms

Numerous microorganisms inhabit the oral cavity, and many bacteria produce acids as a by-product of their metabolism, thereby lowering the intraoral pH. Ingested foodstuffs and liquids can also rapidly change the pH of the mouth, shifting it from mildly alkaline to strongly acidic. In addition, oral biofilms formed on the tooth surfaces following exposure to saliva, bacteria, and food can degrade components in dental restorations, thus exposing different constituents of the restoration. In most cases, the integrity of the restoration is challenged by multispecies oral biofilms that may lead to secondary caries and restoration failure. Thus, bacteria contribute to the alteration of the restorative materials' biocompatibility through production of lactic acid, which lowers the pH, promoting hydrolysis of restorative materials, and through secretion of esterases that further hydrolyze the restoration (Spencer et al., 2014). This cascade results not only in degradation of the material, but also in surface topographical changes, which provoke more biofilm attachment that may lead to restoration failure.

5.5 Enzymes

Enzymes that contribute to the breakdown of restorative materials are not only present in bacteria but are also found in saliva, mineralized dentin, and the dentinal fluid. These endopeptidases include matrix metalloproteinases (MMPs) and cysteine cathepsins, which are collectively responsible for the hydrolytic degradation of extracellular matrix components, such as the adhesive hybrid layer under composite restorations (Mazzoni et al., 2015).

The combination of these chemical, mechanical and thermal challenges is often synergistic. The restorative material is subjected to a variety of fluids at varying temperatures during its lifetime. It is therefore obvious that, over long periods, the effects of these challenges will profoundly influence the material's characteristics and, consequently, the restoration's performance and longevity (Fig. 5.1).

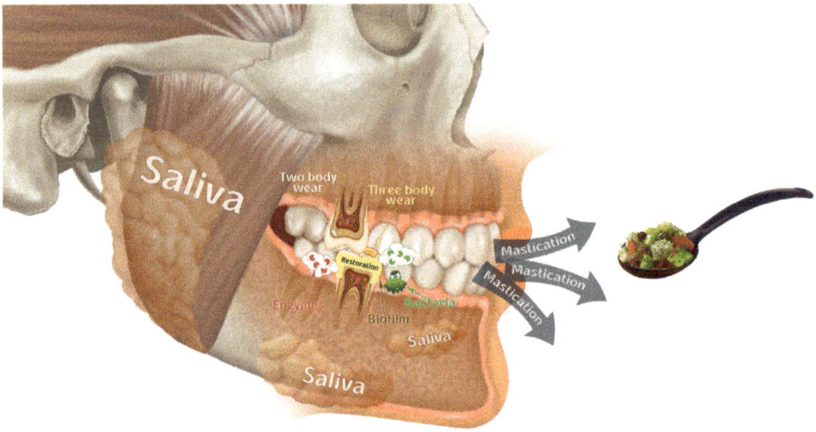

Figure 5.1 Harsh oral cavity environment conditions. *Mastication*: constant stress and strain during mastication. Contacting surfaces cause wear: two-body wear (tooth to tooth) and three-body wear (teeth and food). *Saliva*: the fluid layer between the sliding surfaces, acting as a protective barrier and buffer or a potential source of enzymes. *Microorganisms*: bacteria produce acids lowering the intraoral pH; microorganisms colonize in a dense mass forming biofilm. *Enzymes*: bacterial, salivary, and dentinal enzymes contribute to the breakdown of restorative materials. Illustration by Orit Yeshayahu.

5.6 Amalgam restorations

Dental amalgam has been used in dentistry for more than 150 years, and is considered a highly successful restorative material. Its relatively low cost, low technique sensitivity, high compressive strength, and good wear resistance contribute to its success. During the past century, dental amalgam restorations have been controversial, especially owing to their hazardous mercury content (Wahl and Swift, 2013). Consequently, there is a worldwide trend towards replacing amalgam restorations with mercury-free, adhesive, and tooth-colored materials. Still, a meta-analysis of resin composite restoration function in posterior teeth demonstrated higher rates of secondary caries and decreased longevity compared with posterior amalgam restorations (Moraschini et al., 2015).

Despite the shift towards tooth-colored filling materials, many amalgam restorations are still being placed throughout the world and many more are already present in patients' mouths (Roberts and Charlton, 2009). For decades, set amalgam was considered an inert material that does not release mercury. However, studies in the 1970s and 1980s determined that this was not accurate. Several investigations concluded that daily human mercury exposure from amalgam is about 1 μ g/day from mercury vapor inhalation, and 1 μ g/day from the ingestion of ionic forms (Ekstrand et al., 1998). Despite these findings, this issue remains controversial and evidence supporting the removal of amalgam restorations is still lacking (Lian and Meletis, 1996).

Furthermore, although the number of amalgam restorations was positively correlated with subjects' serum mercury levels, no association was found between the levels and symptoms, including incidence of diabetes, stroke, cancer, and myocardial infarction (Ahlqwist et al., 1999).

During mastication, dental amalgam is subjected to corrosion in the oral environment and to a constant wear process when the restored surfaces contact opposing surfaces. The restoration is affected by masticatory forces originating in the antagonist teeth and in the food being chewed. However, when reviewing in vivo and in vitro corrosion of dental amalgams, no reports of major corrosion products, which includes mercury, are found in the literature. Regardless of the specific amalgam composition, mercury eluted into an aqueous medium is either released into solution or reamalgamated with residual alloys (Okabe, 1987). Dental amalgam is known for its high wear resistance which, although difficult to evaluate, especially in vivo, has been used as the gold standard when evaluating new resin composite materials (Lazaridou et al., 2015).

Mercury release from amalgam under dynamic conditions depends on the acidity of the environment. At extremely low pH values, mercury release was significantly higher than in deionized water. However, it was shown that release from amalgam can be reduced by formation of a tin oxide film on the surface of the mercury-rich gamma 1 phase (Okabe et al., 2003).

Bleaching procedures, using low pH materials were tested in a pilot clinical study, by Cakir et al. (2015) to determine mercury release from amalgam fillings and antioxidant enzyme activity (superoxide dismutase and catalase) in blood, urine, and saliva, after exposure to two different vital tooth-bleaching systems. It was found that either office or home bleaching did not have any effect on the amount of mercury released from amalgam fillings in blood, urine, or saliva, or on the antioxidant-enzyme activities measured in the blood (Cakir et al., 2015).

The average longevity of amalgam restorations in the oral environment is 5–12 years. The main reasons for the failure of amalgam restorations are secondary caries, fracture, marginal deficiencies, wear, and postoperative sensitivity (Lai et al., 2013).

Despite the controversy about the use of amalgam, the World Dental Federation maintain that dental amalgam has a well-documented history of safety and efficacy (Moncada, 2015).

5.7 Resin composite restorations

Composite restorative materials represent a wide family of tooth-colored biomaterials, used to replace missing tooth tissues due to decay, trauma, or congenital reasons.

The use of resin-based restorative materials is increasing, replacing the traditional dental amalgam (Kelly and Smales, 2004; Mitchell et al., 2007; Roulet, 1997) due to its involvement in environmental pollution, potential patient and dental staff health hazards, and its esthetic compromises.

Despite the growing market for dental composites, their safety and biocompatibility are under continuous scrutiny. The increasing awareness of the hazards to patients due to exposure to harmful substances in dental materials is relevant to resin composite materials as well (Geurtsen, 2000).

All dental composites are composed of a polymeric matrix, typically a dimethacrylate resin, reinforcing fillers often made from radiopaque glass, a silane-coupling agent for binding the filler to the matrix, and chemicals that promote or modulate the polymerization reaction (Ferracane, 2011).

Resin-based filling materials may release various components after placement of the restoration. These components include nonpolymerized monomer, filler, and additives, which may be released initially due to incomplete polymerization, and later due to degradation (Van Landuyt et al., 2011).

The polymerization of dimethacrylates passes through two routes: chemical or visible light initiated. Light curing is preferable owing to the finer control of the entire polymerization process (Sideridou et al., 2002). However, full conversion can never be achieved, resulting in the presence of free monomers. Unfortunately, the resin composite materials available today show a degree of conversion varying between 40% and 70% (Kildal and Ruyter, 1994), with an even lower degree of polymerization immediately after light curing (Feng et al., 2009). Release of filler particles or ions such as strontium, fluoride, and aluminum is mainly due to mechanical wear such as mastication, brushing, and parafunction. Little is known regarding the biocompatibility of the filler component (Van Landuyt et al., 2011).

Among the possible components released from resin-based dental materials, nonpolymerized monomers are potentially the most alarming. There is evidence to the effect that monomers may have cytotoxic (Moharamzadeh et al., 2008; Schweikl et al., 2006; Reichl et al., 2001), genotoxic (Geurtsen and Leyhausen, 2001; Lee et al., 2006; Urcan et al., 2010), and allergenic (Arenholt-Bindslev, 1998; Sandberg et al., 2002; Schedle et al., 2007) effects.

The filler component of dental composite consists of various inorganic substances such as glass or quartz (Anusavice, 2003). The filler components improve the physical properties, reduce shrinkage, and increase radio-opacity.

The oral environment places a variety of constraints on the composites. Chemical, mechanical, and microbial conditions challenge the material in different ways with various consequences. A study of the influence of the level of filler loading on the wear resistance of a composite produced inconsistent results (Hu et al., 2003). Presently, the common trend is to minimize filler size and maximize its content to optimize the dental composite requirements (Ferracane, 1995). Attempts have been made to calculate the quantity of constituents released from resin composite restorations: the quantity of substance released related to the oral challenge by estimating total tooth surface area and volume, and the mean size of standard composite restorations (Van Landuyt et al., 2011). It was found that a predictable estimation of the released quantities was possible based on the average size of the restoration.

It might be assumed that the repeated loading, and the wear due to mastication, tooth brushing, and parafunction, would reduce the biocompatibility of dental resin composites, but to date no clear connection has been established (Van Landuyt et al., 2011).

Resin composites absorb water and elute unreacted monomers in an aqueous environment. The water causes silane hydrolysis and formation of microcracks, thus weakening the composite (Oysaed and Ruyter, 1986a,b). The extent and rate of water uptake is dependent upon the density of the polymer network and the potential for hydrogen bonding and polar interactions (Ferracane, 2006). Lower density of the polymer can cause water infiltration and release toxic components.

The most frequently used resin in dental composite combines bisphenol A glycol dimethacrylate (*bis*-GMA) and triethylene glycol dimethacrylate (TEGDMA). *Bis*-GMA possesses a high viscosity rate, TEGDMA is used to lower this rate and achieve a workable viscosity (Sideridou et al., 2004).

Water sorption, solubility, and the behavior of resin composites in the oral aqueous environment have been widely investigated. Venz and Dickens (1991) reported differences in the solubility of different monomers: TEGDMA > *bis*-GMA>Urethane dimethacrylate (UDMA)>N-methyl-l-(3,4-methylenedioxyphenyl)-3-butanamine (HMDMA). Sideridou et al. (2003) compared the water sorption of four different monomers and showed that the order of water sorption of the monomers was TEGDMA>*bis*-GMA>UDMA>*bis*-EMA(4) (ethoxylated bisphenol A glycol dimethacrylate), although the release of the unreacted monomer (*bis*-EMA(4)>*bis*-GMA/UDMA>TEGDMA) did not correlate with the order of water sorption.

In their meta-analysis, Van Landuyt et al. (2011) found that 25 different eluates were released into the oral cavity. The monomers, as part of the polymer matrix, are the most researched and measured component, whereas additives and/or initiators or inhibitors have barely been investigated, although their components can be hazardous.

Enzymes are biological catalysts that accelerate biological reactions such as resin composite degradation. Human saliva contains various enzymes, among them esterases (Lindqvist and Augustinsson, 1975) and MMPs (Delaviz et al., 2014), acetylcholinesterase and pseudocholinesterase being the two main types. Esterases cause degradation of one of the most common monomers used in dental composites and adhesives, 2,2-[4(2-hydroxy 3-methacryloxypropoxy)-phenyl] propane (*bis*-GMA), to form the degradation product 2,2-*bis* [4 (2,3-hydroxy-propoxy)phenyl] propane (*bis*-HPPP) (Finer and Santerre, 2004; Gopferich, 1996; Shokati et al., 2010).

Bisphenol A and bisphenol A dimethacrylate (BIS-DMA) are components found in the resin matrix which are considered to have estrogenic features (Olea et al., 1996) that may affect various endocrine activities (Soderholm and Mariotti, 1999). Estrogen regulates hormonal activity mainly in women, and includes development, growth, and maintenance of secondary sex characteristics.

Research assessing the effects of the components released from the composite matrix is focused mainly on cell cultures and animals. The available data (Soderholm and Mariotti, 1999) from these studies suggest that the amount of bisphenol A formed is inconsequential, and the risk to humans is yet to be proved. However caution must be taken when using dental composites, i.e., following the clinical guidelines for the use of a specific material, isolating the teeth, and polymerizing the composite.

MMPs are another type of enzyme present in human saliva that are secreted from various cells (Delaviz et al., 2014). MMPs are involved in different metabolic and cell processes, that cause degradation of the layer between the resin composite and the tooth, better known as the hybrid layer. Attack on the hybrid layer potentially can lead to microleakage of bacteria, possibly causing secondary caries.

MMPs can be activated by a low pH produced by self-etch and etch-and-rinse adhesives (Zhang and Kern, 2009). Consequently, MMPs compromise the stability of the composite-dentin structure and may contribute to the caries process (Chaussain-Miller et al., 2006).

Cysteine cathepsins are collagen-degrading enzymes that are expressed by odontoblasts (Tersariol et al., 2010). These enzymes, like the MMPS are activated during acid etching or by acid produced by oral microorganisms.

One of the disadvantages of resin composite materials is that plaque tends to build up more frequently on such restorations compared with other restoration materials (Skjorland, 1973; Svanberg et al., 1990), causing gingival irritation and possible recurrent caries. Beyth et al. (2007) showed complete inhibition of *S. mutans* in amalgam in comparison with a minimal effect of resin composite on inhibition of bacterial growth. The bacteria–composite surface interaction causes changes in the roughness of composites which, in turn, may further accelerate biofilm accumulation (Beyth et al., 2008). Other studies report that release of Ethylene glycol dimethacrylate (EGDMA) and TEGDMA from resin composites should be minimized due to their stimulatory effect on the growth of caries-associated microorganisms (Hansel et al., 1998).

In endodontically treated teeth, increased plaque accumulation on the composite core, in addition to the loss of sensation that occurs following root canal treatment, increases the likelihood of secondary caries formation that can lead to the failure of the root canal (Merdad et al., 2010).

One way to deal with bacterial accumulation on resin-based composites is to add antibacterials such as antibiotics, chlorhexidine (Merdad et al., 2010), fluoride (Kohnen and Jansen, 1995), and silver ions (Medlin, 1997) to the composites. Some of these are gradually released, resulting in a decrease in the mechanical properties of the restorative material, inconsistent agent release, or short-term effectiveness, and possible toxicity to the host tissues (Kohnen and Jansen, 1995; Medlin, 1997; Nohr and Macdonald, 1994; Shearer et al., 2000).

An alternative group of antibacterial agents includes polymeric antimicrobials. These can be chemically bound to the base material and thus undergo improved integration (Kawabata and Nishiguchi, 1988). Consequently, polymeric agents have the advantage of being chemically stable and thus may be less toxic to the surrounding tissues.

The esthetics of resin-based composites are excellent, their wear resistance, polishability, and biological properties improving exponentially owing to continuous and worldwide research and development. However, several problems remain regarding the biocompatibility of the resin-based composites.

5.8 Glass-ionomer cement restorations

Glass-ionomer cement (GIC) are favored restorative materials owing to their ease of use and unique biocompatibility, attributable to their good adhesion (Yip et al., 2001). Leakage appears to be largely prevented and, thus, invasion of bacteria at the tooth-filling interface is minimized.

Leaching of component materials may be an advantage in the use of glass ionomers. When they serve as a luting agent or a restorative material, fluoride is released slowly, thereby inhibiting caries formation at the margins of the restorations (Yip et al., 2001). A recent study investigated the cytotoxicity of different restorative glass ionomer materials in relation to the release of incorporated ions such as fluoride, aluminum, and strontium (Kanjevac et al., 2012) and identified that high levels of released fluoride, but not of the other ions, correlated with high levels of cytotoxicity to pulp stem cells. A similar study, testing the effect of released nanoparticles from GIC, showed that incorporation of nanoparticles such as titanium dioxide (TiO_2) in the GICs to improve their mechanical and antibacterial properties, could be harmful systemically when they leached out during function (Garcia-Contreras et al., 2014).

The long-term mechanical properties of GIC are generally tested in the laboratory under simulated oral conditions. The intraoral behavior of restorative materials is a complex process in which mastication occurs in a chemically active environment, resulting in degradation of the restoration. Over time, the deterioration is described in general terms of wear, marginal breakdown, and fatigue fracture owing to cyclic loading (Braem et al., 1994). The deterioration causes material loss from the restoration, with a high risk of toxicity.

In dentistry, the loss of material owing to nonantagonistic contacts has been defined as occlusal contact-free area wear, stemming from material loss by direct contact of an antagonist with the restorative material. The restorative materials are measured experimentally and compared with amalgam as standard (Pelka et al., 1996). GIC exhibits a contact-free area wear five-times greater than amalgam and three-times greater than resin composite materials (Folwaczny et al., 2001). However, despite its well-suited surface wear characteristics, some GIC restorations undergo sudden failure owing to mechanical fatigue (Davidson, 2006).

Tooth structure and restorative materials in the mouth expand upon heating by hot foods and beverages, and contract when exposed to cold substances. Such expansions and contractions may break the marginal seal of an inlay or other tooth fillings, particularly if there is a large difference in the coefficient of thermal expansion between the tooth and the restorative material. Within a practically relevant temperature range between 20°C and 60°C, materials such as resinous composites and amalgam expand more than the tooth tissue, whereas porcelain and glass ionomer cements are well adapted to tooth tissue. The fact that GIC is unaffected by thermal changes occurring during meals contributes to the material's stability and biocomptability.

Recently there has been an improvement in the physical properties of GIC, reducing its deterioration. This improvement together with its low cytotoxicity contribute to the growing use of GIC as a restorative material.

5.9 Summary

Dental restorative materials interact continuously with the oral environment. From the time of placement they are subjected to constant degradation, both mechanical and chemical. One cannot assume that the placed restoration material remains stable during function. On the contrary, it undergoes relentless change.

Mastication wears restorative materials through two- and three-body wear, releasing substances into the oral milieu. Simultaneously, saliva ingredients degrade the restoration while bacteria promote hydrolysis and surface changes. Shifts in temperature change material dimensions, thus also contributing to restoration breakdown.

All of the common restorative materials are subjected to these changes: amalgam metal alloy undergoes acidic corrosion, resin-based filling materials may release nonpolymerized monomer, filler, and additives, due to both incomplete polymerization and degradation, and glass ionomers appear to leak minimally, though the slow fluoride release may be advantageous.

When addressing the question of biocompatibility, the clinician should consider the properties of the materials in the hostile oral environment, rather than the inert material itself, taking into account that all dental materials keep on changing and reacting while functioning.

References

Aguirre, A., Mendoza, B., Levine, M.J., Hatton, M.N., Douglas, W.H., 1989. In vitro characterization of human salivary lubrication. Arch. Oral Biol. 34, 675–677.

Ahlqwist, M., Bengtsson, C., Lapidus, L., Gergdahl, I.A., Schutz, A., 1999. Serum mercury concentration in relation to survival, symptoms, and diseases: results from the prospective population study of women in Gothenburg, Sweden. Acta Odontol. Scand. 57, 168–174.

Anusavice, K., 2003. Phillips' Science of Dental Materials, 11th ed. Saunders, St. Louis, MO.

Arenholt-Bindslev, D., 1998. Environmental aspects of dental filling materials. Eur. J. Oral Sci. 106, 713–720.

Beyth, N., Domb, A.J., Weiss, E.I., 2007. An in vitro quantitative antibacterial analysis of amalgam and composite resins. J. Dent. 35, 201–206.

Beyth, N., Bahir, R., Matalon, S., Domb, A.J., Weiss, E.I., 2008. Streptococcus mutans biofilm changes surface-topography of resin composites. Dent. Mater. 24, 732–736.

Braem, M., Lambrechts, P., Vanherle, G., 1994. Clinical relevance of laboratory fatigue studies. J. Dent. 22, 97–102.

Cakir, F.Y., Ergin, E., Gurgan, S., Sabuncuoglu, S., Arpa, C.S., Tokgoz, I., et al., 2015. Effect of bleaching on mercury release from amalgam fillings and antioxidant enzyme activities: a pilot study. J. Esthet. Restorative Dent. 27, 29–36.

Chaussain-Miller, C., Fioretti, F., Goldberg, M., Menashi, S., 2006. The role of matrix metalloproteinases (MMPs) in human caries. J. Dent. Res. 85, 22–32.

Davidson, C.L., 2006. Advances in glass-ionomer cements. J. Appl. Oral Sci. 14, 3–9.

Delaviz, Y., Finer, Y., Santerre, J.P., 2014. Biodegradation of resin composites and adhesives by oral bacteria and saliva: a rationale for new material designs that consider the clinical environment and treatment challenges. Dent. Mater. 30, 16–32.

Ekstrand, J., Bjorkman, L., Edlund, C., Sandborgh-Englund, G., 1998. Toxicological aspects on the release and systemic uptake of mercury from dental amalgam. Eur. J. Oral Sci. 106, 678–686.

Feng, L., Carvalho, R., Suh, B.I., 2009. Insufficient cure under the condition of high irradiance and short irradiation time. Dent. Mater. 25, 283–289.

Ferracane, J.L., 1995. Current trends in dental composites. Crit. Rev. Oral Biol. Med. 6, 302–318.

Ferracane, J.L., 2006. Hygroscopic and hydrolytic effects in dental polymer networks. Dent. Mater. 22, 211–222.

Ferracane, J.L., 2011. Resin composite—state of the art. Dent. Mater. 27, 29–38.

Finer, Y., Santerre, J.P., 2004. Salivary esterase activity and its association with the biodegradation of dental composites. J. Dent. Res. 83, 22–26.

Folwaczny, M., Mehl, A., Kunzelmann, K.H., Hickel, R., 2001. Clinical performance of a resin-modified glass-ionomer and a compomer in restoring non-carious cervical lesions. 5-year results. Am. J. Dent. 14, 153–156.

Garcia-Contreras, R., Scougall-Vilchis, R.J., Contreras-Bulnes, R., Kanda, Y., Nakajima, H., Sakagami, H., 2014. Effects of TiO2 nano glass ionomer cements against normal and cancer oral cells. In Vivo 28, 895–907.

Geurtsen, W., 2000. Biocompatibility of resin-modified filling materials. Crit. Rev. Oral Biol. Med. 11, 333–355.

Geurtsen, W., Leyhausen, G., 2001. Chemical-biological Interactions of the resin monomer triethyleneglycol-dimethacrylate (TEGDMA). J. Dent. Res. 80, 2046–2050.

Gopferich, A., 1996. Mechanisms of polymer degradation and erosion. Biomaterials 17, 103–114.

Hansel, C., Leyhausen, G., Mai, U.E., Geurtsen, W., 1998. Effects of various resin composite (co)monomers and extracts on two caries-associated micro-organisms in vitro. J. Dent. Res. 77, 60–67.

Hatton, M.N., Loomis, R.E., Levine, M.J., Tabak, L.A., 1985. Masticatory lubrication. The role of carbohydrate in the lubricating property of a salivary glycoprotein-albumin complex. Biochem. J. 230, 817–820.

Hu, X., Marquis, P.M., Shortall, A.C., 2003. Influence of filler loading on the two-body wear of a dental composite. J. Oral Rehab. 30, 729–737.

Kanjevac, T., Milovanovic, M., Volarevic, V., Lukic, M.L., Arsenijevic, N., Markovic, D., et al., 2012. Cytotoxic effects of glass ionomer cements on human dental pulp stem cells correlate with fluoride release. Med. Chem. 8, 40–45.

Kawabata, N., Nishiguchi, M., 1988. Antibacterial activity of soluble pyridinium-type polymers. Appl. Environ. Microbiol. 54, 2532–2535.

Kelly, P.G., Smales, R.J., 2004. Long-term cost-effectiveness of single indirect restorations in selected dental practices. Br. Dent. J. 196, 639–643. discussion 27.

Kildal, K.K., Ruyter, I.E., 1994. How different curing methods affect the degree of conversion of resin-based inlay/onlay materials. Acta Odontol. Scand. 52, 315–322.

Kohnen, W., Jansen, B., 1995. Polymer materials for the prevention of catheter-related infections. Zentralbl. Bakteriol. 283, 175–186.

Lai, G.Y., Zhu, L.K., Li, M.Y., Wang, J., 2013. An in vitro study on the secondary caries-prevention properties of three restorative materials. J. Prosth. Dent. 110, 363–368.

Lazaridou, D., Belli, R., Petschelt, A., Lohbauer, U., 2015. Are resin composites suitable replacements for amalgam? A study of two-body wear. Clin. Oral Investig. 19, 1485–1492.

Lee, D.H., Lim, B.S., Lee, Y.K., Ahn, S.J., Yang, H.C., 2006. Involvement of oxidative stress in mutagenicity and apoptosis caused by dental resin monomers in cell cultures. Dent. Mater. 22, 1086–1092.

Lian, K., Meletis, E.I., 1996. Corrosion of amalgams under sliding wear. Dent. Mater. 12, 146–153.

Lindqvist, L., Augustinsson, K.B., 1975. Esterases in human saliva. Enzyme 20, 277–291.

Mandel, I.D., 1987. The functions of saliva. J. Dent. Res. 66 Spec No: 623-7.

Mazzoni, A., Tjaderhane, L., Checchi, V., Di Lenarda, R., Salo, T., Tay, F.R., et al., 2015. Role of dentin MMPs in caries progression and bond stability. J. Dent. Res. 94, 241–251.

Medlin, J., 1997. Germ warfare. Environ. Health Perspect. 105, 290–292.

Merdad, K., Sonbul, H., Gholman, M., Reit, C., Birkhed, D., 2010. Evaluation of the caries profile and caries risk in adults with endodontically treated teeth. Oral Surg. Oral Med. Oral Pathol. Oral Radiol. Endod. 110, 264–269.

Mitchell, R.J., Koike, M., Okabe, T., 2007. Posterior amalgam restorations—usage, regulation, and longevity. Dent. Clin. North Am. 51, 573–589.

Moharamzadeh, K., Brook, I.M., Scutt, A.M., Thornhill, M.H., Van Noort, R., 2008. Mucotoxicity of dental composite resins on a tissue-engineered human oral mucosal model. J. Dent. 36, 331–336.

Moncada, G., 2015. Seal, replacement or monitoring amalgam restorations with occlusal marginal defects? Results of a 10-year clinical trial. J. Dent. 43 (11), 1371–1378.

Moraschini, V., Fai, C.K., Alto, R.M., Dos Santos, G.O., 2015. Amalgam and resin composite longevity of posterior restorations: a systematic review and meta-analysis. J. Dent. 43, 1043–1050.

Nohr, R.S., Macdonald, J.G., 1994. New biomaterials through surface segregation phenomenon: new quaternary ammonium compounds as antibacterial agents. J. Biomater. Sci. Polymer Ed. 5, 607–619.

Okabe, T., 1987. Mercury in the structure of dental amalgam. Dent. Mater. 3, 1–8.

Okabe, T., Elvebak, B., Carrasco, L., Ferracane, J.L., Keanini, R.G., Nakajima, H., 2003. Mercury release from dental amalgams into continuously replenished liquids. Dent. Mater. 19, 38–45.

Olea, N., Pulgar, R., Perez, P., Olea-Serrano, F., Rivas, A., Novillo-Fertrell, A., et al., 1996. Estrogenicity of resin-based composites and sealants used in dentistry. Environ. Health Perspect. 104, 298–305.

Oysaed, H., Ruyter, I.E., 1986a. Composites for use in posterior teeth: mechanical properties tested under dry and wet conditions. J. Biomed. Mater. Res. 20, 261–271.

Oysaed, H., Ruyter, I.E., 1986b. Water sorption and filler characteristics of composites for use in posterior teeth. J. Dent. Res. 65, 1315–1318.

Pelka, M., Ebert, J., Schneider, H., Kramer, N., Petschelt, A., 1996. Comparison of two- and three-body wear of glass-ionomers and composites. Eur. J. Oral Sci. 104, 132–137.

Reichl, F.X., Durner, J., Hickel, R., Kunzelmann, K.H., Jewett, A., Wang, M.Y., et al., 2001. Distribution and excretion of TEGDMA in guinea pigs and mice. J. Dent. Res. 80, 1412–1415.

Roberts, H.W., Charlton, D.G., 2009. The release of mercury from amalgam restorations and its health effects: a review. Oper. Dent. 34, 605–614.

Roulet, J.F., 1997. Benefits and disadvantages of tooth-coloured alternatives to amalgam. J. Dent. 25, 459–473.

Sandberg, E., Bergenholtz, G., Eklund, C., Dahlgren, U.I., 2002. HEMA bound to self-protein promotes auto-antibody production in mice. J. Dent. Res. 81, 633–636.

Schedle, A., Ortengren, U., Eidler, N., Gabauer, M., Hensten, A., 2007. Do adverse effects of dental materials exist? What are the consequences, and how can they be diagnosed and treated? Clin. Oral Implants Res. 18 (Suppl. 3), 232–256.

Schweikl, H., Spagnuolo, G., Schmalz, G., 2006. Genetic and cellular toxicology of dental resin monomers. J. Dent. Res. 85, 870–877.

Shearer, A.E., Paik, J.S., Hoover, D.G., Haynie, S.L., Kelley, M.J., 2000. Potential of an antibacterial ultraviolet-irradiated nylon film. Biotechnol. Bioeng. 67, 141–146.

Shokati, B., Tam, L.E., Santerre, J.P., Finer, Y., 2010. Effect of salivary esterase on the integrity and fracture toughness of the dentin-resin interface. J. Biomed. Mater. Res. B. Appl. Biomater. 94, 230–237.

Sideridou, I., Tserki, V., Papanastasiou, G., 2002. Effect of chemical structure on degree of conversion in light-cured dimethacrylate-based dental resins. Biomaterials 23, 1819–1829.

Sideridou, I., Tserki, V., Papanastasiou, G., 2003. Study of water sorption, solubility and modulus of elasticity of light-cured dimethacrylate-based dental resins. Biomaterials 24, 655–665.

Sideridou, I., Achilias, D.S., Spyroudi, C., Karabela, M., 2004. Water sorption characteristics of light-cured dental resins and composites based on Bis-EMA/PCDMA. Biomaterials 25, 367–376.

Skjorland, K.K., 1973. Plaque accumulation on different dental filling materials. Scand. J. Dent. Res. 81, 538–542.

Soderholm, K.J., Mariotti, A., 1999. BIS-GMA—based resins in dentistry: are they safe? J. Am. Dent. Assoc. 130, 201–209.

Spencer, P., Ye, Q., Misra, A., Goncalves, S.E., Laurence, J.S., 2014. Proteins, pathogens, and failure at the composite-tooth interface. J. Dent. Res. 93, 1243–1249.

Svanberg, M., Mjor, I.A., Orstavik, D., 1990. Mutans streptococci in plaque from margins of amalgam, composite, and glass-ionomer restorations. J. Dent. Res. 69, 861–864.

Tersariol, I.L., Geraldeli, S., Minciotti, C.L., Nascimento, F.D., Paakkonen, V., Martins, M.T., et al., 2010. Cysteine cathepsins in human dentin-pulp complex. J. Endod. 36, 475–481.

Urcan, E., Scherthan, H., Styllou, M., Haertel, U., Hickel, R., Reichl, F.X., 2010. Induction of DNA double-strand breaks in primary gingival fibroblasts by exposure to dental resin composites. Biomaterials 31, 2010–2014.

Van Landuyt, K.L., Nawrot, T., Geebelen, B., De Munck, J., Snauwaert, J., Yoshihara, K., et al., 2011. How much do resin-based dental materials release? A meta-analytical approach. Dent. Mater. 27, 723–747.

Venz, S., Dickens, B., 1991. NIR-spectroscopic investigation of water sorption characteristics of dental resins and composites. J. Biomed. Mater. Res. 25, 1231–1248.

Wahl, M.J., Swift Jr., E.J., 2013. Critical appraisal: dental amalgam update—part II: biological effects. J. Esthet. Restorative Dent. 25, 433–437.

Yip, H.K., Tay, F.R., Ngo, H.C., Smales, R.J., Pashley, D.H., 2001. Bonding of contemporary glass ionomer cements to dentin. Dent. Mater. 17, 456–470.

Zhang, S.C., Kern, M., 2009. The role of host-derived dentinal matrix metalloproteinases in reducing dentin bonding of resin adhesives. Inter. J. Oral Sci. 1, 163–176.

Biocompatibility of luting cements for dental applications

6

C.H. Pameijer
Emeritus Professor, University of Connecticut, Farmington, CT, United States

Abstract

Fixed crown and bridgework consists of multiple critical procedures, of which the final step, the selection of a luting agent for permanent cementation, represents a particularly difficult choice due to the large number of cements that are available. A proper choice is further complicated by the large variety in physical and other properties, as well as by the composition of the substrate to be cemented. The most frequently asked question by practitioners relates to retention, while it should focus on biocompatibility. The first is controlled by the practitioner, adhering to the principles of crown preparation (i.e., total angle of convergence, preparation height and, if needed, auxiliary grooves or boxes), while the latter is determined by the properties of the material and affects postcementation and long-term service and comfort to patients.

This chapter aims to discuss composition and the biocompatibility of commercially available cements. The following cements will be discussed: liners and bases, temporary cements and permanent cements (i.e., zinc phosphate cement, polycarboxylate cement, glass ionomer cement, resin cement, resin modified glass ionomer cement, self-etching resin-based cement and a hybrid calcium aluminate/glass ionomer cement). Currently available literature will be quoted to support biocompatibility and postoperative reactions of the various cements.

Biocompatibility testing of luting agents is described in the ISO 7405 and the ANSI/ADA Specification #41, Recommended Standard Practices for Biological Evaluation of Dental Materials. The recent changes in recommendations will be outlined and explained.

Future trends are focused on developing permanent cements that are bioactive in order to seal the restoration–tooth interface, thus preventing bacteria from leaking along the interface causing postoperative sensitivity, secondary decay, and ultimately the demise of the pulp. Finally, information will be provided about the most prevalent dental cements and their manufacturers.

Chapter Outline

Biocompatibility of Dental Biomaterials. DOI: http://dx.doi.org/10.1016/B978-0-08-100884-3.00006-0

6.1 Introduction

Currently, numerous luting agents, or cements as they are usually referred to, are available for the cementation of fixed crowns and bridges, and veneers. Therefore the choice of the most suitable luting agent for a given clinical situation can be a difficult task, even for the most experienced clinician. Restorations made of precious or nonprecious metal, porcelain fused to metal, low- and high-strength ceramics, full or partial coverage, require an understanding of the physical and biological properties and other attributes of both restorative materials and luting agents. This chapter aims at addressing the biocompatibility of currently available luting agents (cements) and how they affect long-term performance and clinical comfort in patients. A wide range of formulations has been developed over the last 100 years, however, in this chapter emphasis will be placed on the contemporary most frequently used cements, whether used for luting or bonding.

6.1.1 Classification of cements

Cements can be classified as follows:

1. liners and bases;
2. temporary (provisional) cements;
3. permanent cements.

6.1.1.1 Liners and bases

The dental profession prefers the use of visible-light-curing materials, in particular resin-modified glass ionomer (RMGI) cements, also referred to as resin reinforced glass ionomer (RRGI), when there is a need for a base or a liner. The reason is based on the fast-setting characteristics by means of visible-light curing. Another important reason for their use arises from the passive application of the material, unlike crown cementation that generates hydraulic pressure, which in the case of acid–base reaction cements can be a contributory factor to pulpal irritation (Pameijer, 1992). Furthermore acid etching of the base material allows for a strong bond with dentin-bonding resins while the adjacent dentin benefits from sustained fluoride release.

Although calcium hydroxide for a base is a good choice, subsequent etching required for a bonded restoration causes disintegration of the material unless a light-curing calcium hydroxide is used. In addition, calcium hydroxide has inferior compressive strength compared to RMGI.

6.1.1.2 Temporary (provisional) cements

The objective of using provisional cements is to retain the provisional restoration and to act as a palliative dressing after the trauma from preparation. For that purpose eugenol-, noneugenol-, resin-, or polycarboxylate-based provisional cements can be used. Caution has to be exercised when using eugenol-containing cements. As not all powder reacts with the eugenol, unreacted eugenol is present after the material has set, which will penetrate into the dentinal tubules (Pameijer and Wendt, 1995). The danger of this is explained below. Eugenol also inhibits the polymerization of resin-based materials subsequently used as liners, bases, bonding agents or permanent restorative filling material. It has been reported that eugenol-containing temporary cements that are used prior to indirect bonding restorations reduce the bond strength of both total- and self-etching adhesive systems to dentin (Ribeiro et al., 2011). However, no differences in bond strengths were observed when using eugenol-free or eugenol-containing provisional cements followed by self-adhesive resin cements by other authors (Bagis et al., 2011).

In spite of this controversy the majority of publications report reduced bond strength of luting agents when eugenol-containing temporary cements are used (Silva et al., 2011; Altintas et al., 2011).

Is it therefore advisable to use noneugenol temporary cements if, during the subsequent treatment, resin-based materials are used? This will depend on the type of cement used. The setting reaction of acid–base reaction cements is not affected by eugenol and therefore they can safely be used. After the trauma from preparation this is an advantage as eugenol at a safe distance from the pulp, >0.75 mm, has palliative properties. However, when the remaining dentin thickness (RDT) to the pulp is less, eugenol becomes more of an irritant. At a distance of less than 0.5 mm eugenol acts as an irritant, which becomes progressively worse with lower RDT, and when in direct contact with the pulp it will cause pulp necrosis (Stanley, 1981). Therefore, the biocompatibility of eugenol-containing temporary cements should be recognized and respected depending on proximity to the pulp, which can only be subjectively estimated, and in context of the choice of permanent cement for the subsequent treatment.

Furthermore, the application of any temporary cement, whether eugenol-containing or not, contaminates the dentin, which may interfere with adhesion (Pameijer, 1992).

6.1.1.3 Permanent cements

The chronological development of luting agents from the late 1800s to the present day is shown in Fig. 6.1. For almost 100 years, only zinc phosphate cement was available; however, technological advances have led to a rapid increase in the number of cements, especially since the 1970s, and today the choice is extensive.

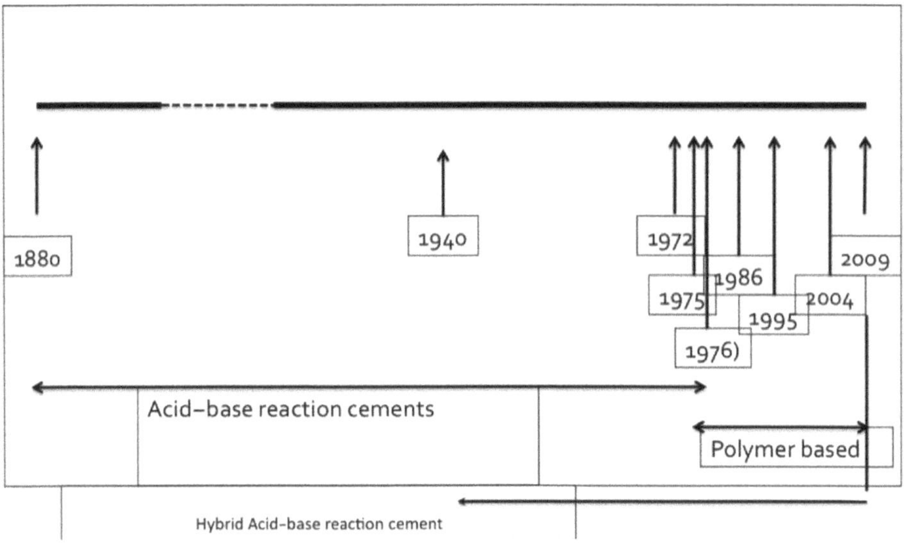

Figure 6.1 Chronological representation of the development of dental luting agents. Note that the increase in the development of new cements since the 1970s was realized by an increase in research and improvements in technology.

Zinc phosphate cement was introduced c.1879, and although the formulation has been refined for more than a century, it is a luting agent that has consistently been successful in clinical practice and even today is still considered the 'gold' standard.

6.1.2 Zinc phosphate cement

This cement sets according to an acid–base reaction and is marketed as a powder/liquid. The basic composition of the powder is zinc oxide with magnesium oxide added as a modifier (±10%) while other oxides such as bismuth and silica may be present to provide radiopacity and as a filler, respectively. Zinc phosphate cement has several favorable physical properties (Anusavice, 1991). Compressive strength of the cement base material compared to zinc oxide and eugenol and calcium hydroxide for instance is much higher. After 24 hours it can reach 104 MPa, while the diametral strength is 5.5 MPa. Another favorable property is the film thickness, which refers to the thickness of the cement between a restoration and the tooth structure. The thickness of this film plays a significant role in the retention of the prosthesis. Film thickness varies with (1) the amount of force applied during seating of a prosthesis, (2) the manner in which the force is applied to the prosthesis during seating, (3) the configuration of the prosthesis relative to its hindering or facilitating the flow of cement, and (4) the fit of the prosthesis on the prepared tooth. The film thickness values reported in the literature typically range from 25 to 150 μm (Anusavice, 1991). Zinc phosphate cement also has a low solubility compared to other cements, 0.06 weight% (Anusavice, 1991).

The liquid is essentially composed of phosphoric acid, water, aluminum phosphate, and sometimes zinc phosphate, and has a very low pH. The water content is approximately 33 ± 5% and is an important factor as it controls the rate and type of powder/liquid reaction (Anusavice, 1991).

When the powder reacts with the liquid a considerable amount of heat is generated (exothermic reaction) and when the mix is complete the cement reaches a pH of 2.14. Since the cement is placed on and in prepared teeth when still in a "wet consistency" as not all liquid has reacted with the powder, unreacted phosphoric acid liquid with a low pH of ±1.5 comes in contact with the preparation and causes an immediate (within 5 seconds) dissolution of the smear layer and smear plugs. Since cementation can cause a considerable amount of hydraulic pressure, the unreacted acid is subsequently squeezed into the dentinal tubules and, depending on the RDT, can cause irritation to the pulp. Therefore, the pulp has to cope with not only heat but low pH as well. The greater the RDT, the more beneficial the buffering action of the fluid in the dentinal tubules is and the less the effect of the acid. Furthermore, a greater RDT also diminishes the thermal effect. When fully reacted after 24 hours, the set cement reaches a pH of 5.5. Since it never becomes neutral it will always exhibit some irritation (Pameijer, 1992). Postcementation hypersensitivity is indeed a frequently occurring clinical problem, which either resolves over time or may result in the need for endodontic treatment. If sensitivity resolves, it is through the protective action of secretion of secondary dentin by odontoblasts, which over time increases the RDT. This process does not start in humans until 3 weeks after the insult has taken place, and deposition of secondary dentin occurs at a rate of micrometers per day (Stanley, 1981). If the pulp cannot cope with the insult, it can become necrotic and then requires root canal treatment. Therefore, although the set luting material may demonstrate many favorable attributes, postcementation discomfort is a known undesirable side effect of this cement, which adversely influences its biocompatibility. Attempts at blocking access of the unreacted phosphoric acid to the dentinal tubules have been made by applying a varnish, Copalite, a natural copal resin in a solvent. Unfortunately, the varnish reduces the retention of the restoration by as much as 50% according to some authors (Felton et al., 1987), as it greatly reduces the micromechanical retention.

To summarize, zinc phosphate cement is a luting agent that demonstrates overall satisfactory biocompatibility providing several precautions are taken into consideration:

1. an accurate powder:liquid ratio;
2. thorough mixing that allows the maximum amount of powder to react with the acid, thus reducing the amount of unreacted acid;
3. a proximity to the pulp that is ideally ≥1 mm;
4. appropriate protection of the pulp if clinical judgment estimates the preparation to be close to the pulp.

6.1.3 Zinc polycarboxylate cement

Polycarboxylate cement also sets according to an acid–base reaction and was introduced by Smith in the 1960s (Smith, 1971). The powder is composed of mainly zinc oxide, magnesium oxide, bismuth, and aluminum oxide. It may also contain stannous fluoride, which increases its strength compared to the original nonfluoride formulation (Greenland, 1974). The liquid is composed of an aqueous solution of polyacrylic acid or a copolymer of acrylic acid and other unsaturated carboxylic acids. Fluoride release by the cement is a small fraction (15–20%) of that released from materials such as silicophosphate and glass ionomer cements (GICs) (Anusavice, 1991). This is an important feature as far as biocompatibility is concerned, as will be explained when GICs are discussed.

When mixed at the recommended powder:liquid ratio, the final mix appears more viscous than zinc phosphate cement. However, the low viscosity can be offset by vibratory action during seating, yielding a film thickness of ±25 μm. At no time should the cement be under-mixed by incorporating less powder to make the viscosity resemble that of zinc phosphate cement, as this will adversely affect the compressive strength, which at 55 MPa is already lower than that of zinc phosphate cement (>~100 MPa). Biocompatibility testing of polycarboxylate cement in subhuman primates demonstrated by means of histology that the cement reacted very favorably and caused no pulpal inflammation of significance, even at an RDT of 0.2 mm (unpublished data). It has been speculated that the long molecular chains of the polyacrylic acid prevent penetration into the dentinal tubules; however, it should be noted that both zinc phosphate and polycarboxylate cements have a low pH immediately after mixing. Polycarboxylate cement (and glass ionomers) exhibits a property called chelation, which is the ability to bond to the Ca ions of the tooth. It is possible that this bond reduces microleakage microorganisms that can cause irritation to the pulp, thus contributing to the cement's biocompatibility.

In summary, the biocompatibility of polycarboxylate cement appears very good; however, as a permanent cement, early washout has caused decementation resulting in failed restorations, either due to improperly mixed cement or the inherent physical properties. Currently, polycarboxylate cements are mostly used for long-term temporary cementation.

6.1.4 Glass ionomer cement

GICs were developed in the early 1970s in the United Kingdom and were first described by Wilson and Kent (1972). GICs set by means of chelation as a result of an acid–base reaction and adhere strongly to enamel and to some extent to dentin. They also release fluoride ions. Initially used as restorative materials, GICs further evolved into luting agents, which is the predominant application of this class of material today.

The powder consists of aluminosilicates with high fluoride content. The material is formed by the fusion of quartz, alumina, cryolite, fluorite, aluminum trifluoride, and aluminum phosphate at temperatures of 1100–1300°C. This glass frit is cooled to a dull glow, quenched in water, and subsequently ground into 45-μm particles.

The liquid is composed of polyacrylic acid and tartaric acid, the latter to accelerate the setting reaction. The reaction of the powder with the liquid causes decomposition, migration, gelation, postsetting hardening, and further slow maturation. The polyacrylic acid reacts with the outer surface of the particles resulting in release of calcium, aluminum, and fluoride ions. When a sufficient amount of metal ions has been released, gelation occurs, and hardening continues for about 24 hours (Wilson and Kent, 1972).

GICs display a relatively low curing shrinkage; within the first 10 minutes 40–50% of shrinkage has occurred. Due to their surface roughness, which promotes plaque accumulation, they were never suitable as a desirable restorative material, except perhaps in pedodontics when fluoride release was thought to help combat decay.

In spite of being promoted as a luting agent demonstrating biocompatibility, the Council of Dental Materials of the American Dental Association received frequent reports of postcementation hypersensitivity. The then-accepted ANSI/ADA Specification 41, Recommended Standard Practices for Biological Evaluation of Dental Materials recommended luting agents to be tested for pulp reactions in nonrodent animals following passive insertion of a more viscous than luting consistency mix in Class V restorations. Histology demonstrated that a GIC tested in primates according to these guidelines elicited no pulpal reaction and was therefore determined to be nonirritating (Pameijer and Stanley, 1988). However, in a subsequent study, also in subhuman primates by means of histological analysis of the pulps, complete crowns were cemented adhering to a clinically more relevant cementation protocol, with a cement mix of normal luting consistency (Pameijer et al., 1991). In this study it was determined that hydraulic pressure generated during crown cementation caused postcementation irritation to the pulp. It was clearly demonstrated that, depending on the RDT, GIC caused pulpal inflammation which, rather than subsiding over time, increased in severity. As a result of this study a change in protocol in the ANSI/ADA Specification 41 was instituted, which now calls for a pressure insertion technique. Rather than using the laborious indirect technique of crown preparation, impressions, and cementing all metal cast crowns as was done in the aforementioned study, Class V composite resin inlays were fabricated and cemented with the experimental GIC. This technique generates hydraulic pressure mimicking complete crown cementation. Furthermore, Class V inlays are usually closer to the pulp than crown preparations and therefore result in a more acute test of biological reactions. Years of studies to determine why GICs cause postcementation hypersensitivity have not resulted in conclusive proof. A convincing case can be made that fluoride, which is actively released from the material, may be responsible for the hypersensitivity. Fluoride is a known irritant (poison), and therefore the closer the proximity to the pulp the greater the irritating effect. Having excluded all other variables over many years of research this author now believes fluoride to be the reason for postoperative sensitivity. To summarize, the biocompatibility of GICs can be managed by taking the following precautions:

1. a sufficient amount of RDT, preferably >1 mm;
2. ideally waiting for a period of 3 weeks between preparation and final cementation, allowing for recovery of the pulp after the trauma of preparation;
3. mechanical mixing of the cement in triturated capsules to ensure an accurate powder:liquid ratio of the final mix;
4. proper isolation of the cement during cementation and afterwards to prevent salivary contamination;
5. using a light-curing dentin bonding resin to protect the margins of the restoration to allow complete setting of the cement, which takes 24 hours, thus preventing weakening of the cement at the most critical area, the cement margin.

6.1.5 Resin cements

As an alternative to acid–base reaction cements, resin cements were introduced in the mid-1980s. Resin cements are polymers to which filler has been added as well as fluoride that set by polymerization of the resin monomers. Polymer degradation due to hydrolysis and a lack of bonding to enamel and dentin make these cements unsuitable as stand-alone luting agents, as it leads to leakage and early failure of the restoration. Additionally, incomplete polymerization can lead to irritation of the pulp by unreacted monomers, which are highly toxic (Goldberg, 2008). However, in combination with a dentin bonding agent, many resin cements have superior properties compared to acid–base reaction cements and are routinely used for the bonding of porcelain laminate veneers to enamel. Understandably there is a reluctance by practitioners to etch complete crown preparations that are on dentin, which is a necessary step for most bonding agents. Even the self-etching dentin bonding agents are not ideal because of concerns regarding postoperative sensitivity. In summary, while fully polymerized resin cements can be considered to demonstrate biocompatibility, without the use of a bonding agent these cements are not recommended for crown and bridge cementation.

6.1.6 Resin-modified glass ionomer

The class of RMGI or RRGI as they are sometimes termed, are cements indicated for the luting of crowns and bridges, as well as inlay and onlay restorations. They are hybrid formulations of resin and glass ionomer components each with their own setting characteristics. The RMGI cements are relatively easy to handle and are suitable for routine application with metal-based crown and bridgework (Bunek and Powers, 2012). However, their use is limited when adhesively cementing ceramics with smooth, nonretentive surfaces (Al-Harbi et al., 2015; Frankenberger et al., 2015; Martins et al., 2015). In addition, adhesion to tooth structure is not strong and was reported to be around 4 MPa (Godoy-Bezerra et al., 2006). Some early formulations have displayed excess water sorption (>2%), causing swelling, frequently resulting in ceramic fracture. Current commercial examples of the RMGI cements include: RelyX Luting, RelyX Luting Plus (3 M/ESPE), Fuji Plus (GC) (GC-America), and UltraCem RRGI Luting Cement (Ultradent Products Inc.).

A review article of the biological effects of RMGI cements in clinical dentistry was published in 2008 (Nicholson and Czarnecka, 2008). Information on RMGIs and on 2-hydroxyethyl methacrylate (HEMA), the most damaging substance released by these materials, was collected from over 50 published papers. HEMA released from these materials causes a variety of damaging biological effects, ranging from pulpal inflammation (Nicholson and Czarnecka, 2008) to allergic contact dermatitis. However, clinical results with RMGI cements are generally favorable. According to the authors, RMGIs cannot be considered to demonstrate biocompatibility to nearly the same extent as conventional glass-ionomers. Care needs to be taken with regard to their use in dentistry and, in particular, dental personnel may be at risk from adverse effects such as contact dermatitis and other immunological responses. Interestingly, RMGIs have a better clinical track record than GICs (Nicholson and Czarnecka, 2008).

In summary, generally few complaints have been reported about postoperative cementation hypersensitivity and typically RMGIs are considered to demonstrate biocompatibility. Yet, RMGIs are in the category of resin cements, therefore water sorption and degradation through hydrolysis are negative features that should not be ignored or underestimated.

At present conflicting data regarding RMGI performance is contradicted by successful clinical use.

6.1.7 Adhesive resin cements

The less than ideal adhesive properties of the RMGIs have led to further development of resin-based luting agents, resulting in the introduction of adhesive resin cements. Compositional changes in monomers, filler, and initiator technology were introduced, leading to adhesive cements that do not require pretreatment or bonding agents to maximize their performance. Examples include: MaxCem (Kerr), RelyX Unicem (3M/ESPE), Breeze (Pentron), Embrace Wet Bond (Pulpdent Corporation) that are popular due to a wide range of applications. Yet in a similar manner to resin and RMGI cements, polymer degradation over time remains an issue. Furthermore, MMPs that are fossilized within mineralized dentin can be released and activated during bonding (Pashley et al., 2004). These endogenous collagenolytic enzymes are on the collagen fibers that are needed for bonding and their slow degrading enzymatic action is beyond the control of even the most meticulous clinician. Reports have appeared that recommend pretreatment of the dentin with 2.0% chlorhexidine gluconate with a pH of 6.0, which prevents the action of the endogenous enzymes (Ricci et al., 2010). One report on biocompatibility appeared in the literature in contrast to the numerous publications on bond strength to various substrates and marginal leakage. This clinical investigation (Blatz et al., 2013) compared a self-adhesive cement (iCem, Heraeus Kulzer) with an RMGI (Fuji Plus, GC-America) and reported that crowns cemented with the self-adhesive cement produced less sensitivity than the control teeth with RMGI. No difference in sensitivity was noted after 24 hours; however, after 3 weeks the self-adhesive cement scored lower sensitivity values. As mentioned previously for resin cements and RMGIs, water sorption resulting in bond degradation is an inherent problem for all resin-based cements (Liu et al., 2011).

6.1.8 Bioactive hybrid-acid-based CaAl/glass ionomer

A recently developed dental luting agent intended for permanent cementation of crowns and bridges, gold inlays and onlays, prefabricated metal crowns, cast post and cores, and all-zirconia or all-alumina crowns has been introduced. Ceramir C&B (Doxa Dental AB, Uppsala, Sweden) is a water-based hybrid composition comprising calcium aluminate and glass ionomer components that is mixed with distilled water. The setting mechanism of Ceramir C&B is a combination of a glass ionomer reaction and an acid–base reaction of the type occurring in hydraulic cements. The incorporation of the calcium aluminate component provides several unique properties compared with conventional GICs. It has been demonstrated that the material has bioactive properties according to the following tests (Lööf et al., 2008). After storage at 37°C in phosphate-buffered saline for 1 hour, 1 day, 7 days, and 4 weeks, samples were analyzed in order to investigate if a surface layer of hydroxyapatite had formed. Technical analysis included grazing incidence X-ray diffraction, scanning electron microscopy, energy dispersive spectroscopy, and transmission electron microscopy.

There are several features that strongly contribute to the biocompatibility profile of the material. These include the fact that immediately after setting the material is slightly acidic, pH 4. After 1 hour the pH is already neutral, and after 3–4 hours the material reaches a basic pH of 8.5 and stays basic throughout its service. This short period of mild acidity is in contrast to other acid–base reaction cements that have a lower initial acidity and after 24 hours remain acidic, the consequences of which have been explained in the previous sections. This basic pH property reached in a matter of hours is the most important feature of the material contributing to its biocompatibility and to the bioactivity, while in addition apatite is created on its surface when in contact with phosphate-containing solutions (Lööf et al., 2008). The apatite forms during hardening but its formation continues when the hardened material is in contact with phosphate solutions through the interaction with calcium aluminate (Jefferies et al., 2015). Additionally, the material produces an excess of Ca^{2+} ions, which also contributes to its bioactivity and ability to remineralize tooth structure. The incorporation of calcium aluminate locks in the GIC structure and hinders the ionomer glass from continuously leaching over time. Therefore the clinical behavior of this material is very different from conventional glass ionomers that leach ions after setting. Ceramir C&B has an initial fluoride release comparable with a glass ionomer, although the release decreases with time. Unique properties such as apatite formation and remineralization develop quickly and continue to be active thus contributing to sealing of the marginal interface and increasing especially enamel margins' resistance against acid attack from bacteria.

To summarize, the biocompatibility of the material appears very good and the literature has reported no postoperative hypersensitivity (Jefferies et al., 2009; Jefferies et al., 2013).

Polycarboxylate cements and Ceramir C&B both demonstrate biocompatibility and are the least irritating cements available today.

6.2 Recommended tests for biocompatibility of dental cements

Tests for biocompatibility are to be conducted either according to the ISO 7405 or the ANSI/ADA Standard # 41, Evaluation of Biocompatibility of Medical Devices used in Dentistry. Currently efforts are in progress to align the ISO 7405 with the ANSI/ADA Standard #41 in order to provide similar global guidelines for the various tests. At present, Standard #41 provides more detailed information about test methods, however. The method for testing dental cements is described in detail and is a clinically relevant test not mentioned in the current ISO 7405. It is anticipated that with the next review both ANSI 7405 and Spec #41 are better aligned and represent mostly similar methodologies.

Each medical device used in dentistry should be subjected to a structured biological evaluation program within a risk management process (see ISO 10993-1). Guidance on the implementation of this program is provided in ISO 14971 and ISO 10993-1. The selection of test methods should be based upon consideration of the intended use of the medical device and the tissue(s) which the medical device may contact, and the duration of the contact. Materials should be tested in vitro and in vivo.

This group below comprises in vitro tests of cytotoxicity, which are among the first tests to be performed before the more definitive and clinically relevant in vivo tests are conducted. General guidance for in vitro cytotoxicity tests is presented in ISO 10993-5. Detailed test protocols for the agar or agarose diffusion and filter diffusion methods, appropriate to dental materials, are included in this International Standard. The in vitro cytotoxicity methods include:

1. agar diffusion test;
2. filter diffusion test;
3. direct contact or extract tests in accordance with ISO 10993-5;
4. dentin barrier cytotoxicity test;
5. tooth slice model.

This list does not indicate that all cytotoxicity tests mentioned above have to be performed for each medical device under consideration.

In order to simulate hydraulic pressure during crown cementation Class V composite resin inlays should be fabricated (Pameijer et al., 1991). Using a direct technique, artificial saliva can be used as a lubricant in the preparation followed by insertion of a light-curing resin composite. After light curing and removal of the resin composite inlay the cavity needs to be thoroughly rinsed and prepared to receive the inlay for final cementation. After insertion the inlay should be held under pressure until the initial set of the cement has occurred, thus simulating the hydraulic forces of full crown cementation (Pameijer and Stanley, 1988). (Note: overfilling of the preparation facilitates inlay removal while the excess can be cut back after cementation following hardening of the luting agent. It is recommended that ample time should be given for the setting reaction to reach completion before removing excess resin composite. A fine diamond high-speed bur and light pressure with copious water cooling is efficient and will prevent unwanted disruption of the integrity of the cement.) In small animals, ensure that the cavities reach into the inner ⅓ of the dentin without exposure of the pulp. Note: it is *not* acceptable to mix a luting agent to a heavier than luting consistency and thus test it as a filling material, as was recommended in the past. When preparing full crowns and to ensure acceptable proximity to the pulp (0.5–1.0mm) it is recommended to first prepare a Class V cavity, essentially serving as a guide to reach the desired proximity to the pulp, followed by completion of the crown preparation.

Fig. 6.2A, B and C show subsequently a Cl V preparation in a canine of a subhuman primate, the overfilled resin composite and extruded cement, and the finished cemented inlay.

6.3 Future developments

RMGI cements or resin-modified cements will most likely dominate in the immediate future as they are easy to handle and find universal application. Emphasis will be placed on developing bioactive cements, whether resin based or of different formulation, with the added benefit that the restoration margins will be sealed and the surrounding tooth structure will be mineralized. A few materials are currently

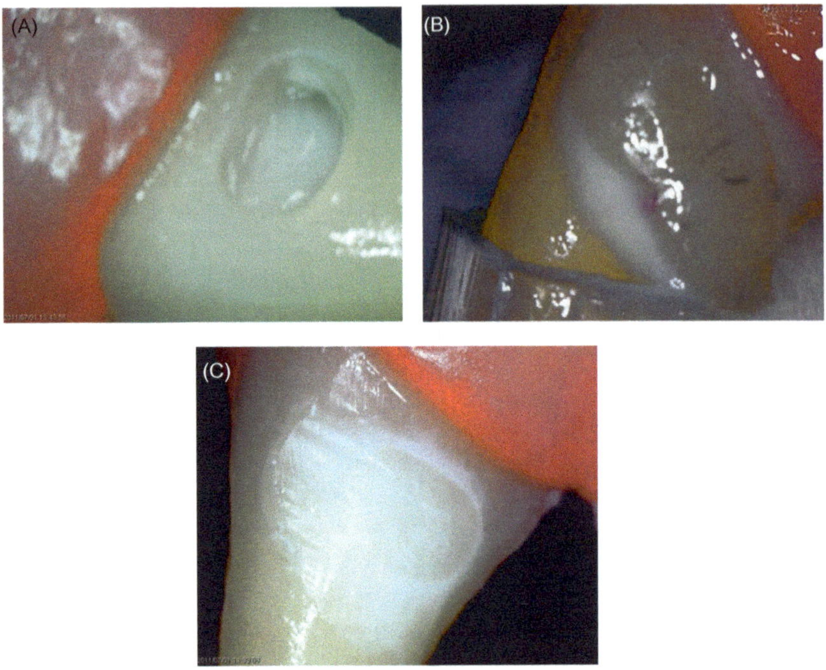

Figure 6.2 (A) Completed Cl V inlay preparation in a canine of a subhuman primate. (B) Extruded cement around the margin of Cl V inlay preparation. (C) Cemented composite inlay after finishing with fine diamonds in a high-speed hand piece and copious water-cooling. Allow for ample setting time before finishing the inlay flush with enamel.

available, Ceramir C&B by Doxa and ACTIVA BioACTIVE RESTORATIVE by Pulpdent Corporation. When Ceramir C&B, a hybrid Ca Aluminate cement, comes in contact with phosphate-containing solutions such as phosphate-buffered saline or saliva, hydroxyapatite formation develops which adheres to the substrate and fills the gap between restoration and tooth, thus sealing the margin and preventing bacteria from entering. This principle has been reported in several publications (Lööf et al., 2008; Jefferies et al., 2013). Bioactivity of cements and restorative materials is a new phenomenon. Strictly speaking and depending on the definition, materials such as calcium hydroxide and mineral trioxide aggregate (MTA), have bioactive properties as well. Calcium hydroxide stimulates the development of preodontoblast and odontoblasts, which results in the formation of reparative dentin. MTA in contact with moisture produces calcium hydroxide and produces the same effect as mentioned above.

Future research will focus on developing bioactive materials for use in restorative dentistry, as well as for the cementation of crown and bridgework.

6.4 Commercially available cements

A list of commercially available cements, their manufacturers and links to their websites is listed in Table 6.1. It is by no means the intention to provide a complete list of all cements that are commercially available.

Table 6.1 **Commercially available cements**

Company	Product	Website
Zinc phosphate cements		
Keystone Industries	Fleck's Zinc Phosphate Cement	www.enamelitellc.com
Bosworth Company	Zinc Phosphate Cement	www.bosworth.com
Polycarboxylate cements		
3M ESPE dental products	Durelon Carboxylate Luting Cement	www.3MESPE.com
Pulpdent Corporation	PolyCarb WaterSet Cement	www.pulpdent.com
Glass ionomer cements		
3M ESPE Dental Products	Ketac Cem Glass Ionomer	www.3MESPE.com
GC America, Inc.	GC Fuji I Glass Ionomer Cement	www.gcamerica.com
Pulpdent Corporation	GlassLute Glass Ionomer Cement	www.pulpdent.com
Resin cement		
L D Caulk & Company	Calibra Esthetic Resin Cement	www.dentsply.com
Pentron	Cement-It Universal C&B	www.pentron.com
Ivoclar Vivadent N.A.	Variolink II	www.ivoclarvivadent.com
Pulpdent Corporation	ResiLute Resin Cement	www.pulpdent.com
Premier Dental Products	IntegraCem Dual Cure Resin Cement	www.premier-dental.com
Pulpdent Corporation	Flows-Rite	www.pulpdent.com
Resin-modified glass ionomer cements		
3M ESPE Dental Products	RelyX Luting Plus Cement RMGI	www.3MESPE.com
GC America, Inc.	GC FujiCEM—RMGI	www.gcamerica.com
Ultradent Products Inc.	UltraCem Resin Reinforced GI cement	www.ultradent.com
Self-adhesive resin cement		
3M ESPE Dental Products	RelyX Unicem 2	www.3MESPE.com
Kerr Mfg Company	Maxcem Elite	www.kerr.com
Pulpdent Corporation	Embrace WetBond Resin cement	www.pulpdent.com
Kuraray America, Inc.	Panavia SA Cement	www.kuraraydental.com
Voco Dental Materials	Bifix SE Luting Cement	www.voco.com/us/company
GC America, Inc.	G-CEM LinkAce Luting Cement	www.gcamerica.com
Pentron	Breeze	www.pentron.com
L D Caulk & Company	SmartCem2	www.dentsply.com
Parkell Products Inc.	C&B Metabond	www.parkell.com
Coltene/Whaledent	ParaBond	www.parkell.com
Shofu Dental Corp	MonoCem	www.shofu.com
Ca Al Hybrid cement		
Doxa Dental AB	CeramirCrown & Bridge Cement	www.doxadental.com

Clinical Indications For Use of Luting Agents

Good Choice = Green
OK = Yellow, but better choices are available
No = Red
DBA = Dentin Bonding Agent NECESSARY. Increases retention and provides a seal.

	1 Single PFM 3-Unit Bridge No Sensitivity During Interim Good Retention	2 Single PFM 3-Unit Bridge Sensitivity During Interim Good Retention	3 Single PFM 3-Unit Bridge No Sensitivity During Interim Poor Retention	4 Single PFM 3-Unit Bridge Sensitivity During Interim Poor Retention	5 Large Bridge No Sensitivity During Interim Good Retention	6 Large Bridge Sensitivity During Interim Good Retention	7 Large Bridge No Sensitivity/ Sensitivity During Interim Poor Retention	8 All Ceramic, Inlay, Onlay, Crown (Pressable)	9 Implant Crown	10 1.Cast P&C 2.Prefab P&C 3.Fiber Post	11 High Strength Ceramics
Zinc Phosphate	OK	NO	NO	NO	OK	NO	NO	NO	OK	1.GoodChoice 2.GoodChoice 3. NO	NO
Glass Ionomer	Good Choice	NO	OK	NO	OK	NO	NO	NO	Good Choice	1.OK 2. OK 3. NO	OK
Resin Cement	Good Choice with DBA	NO	Good Choice with DBA	NO	OK with DBA	NO	NO	Good Choice with DBA	OK	1-3.Good Choice with DBA	OK with DBA
Resin Modified Glass Ionomer	Good Choice	OK	Good Choice	OK	Good Choice	OK	OK	NO	OK	1-3. OK	OK
Self-Etching resin Cement	Good Choice	OK	Good Choice	OK	Good Choice	OK	Good Choice	OK	Good Choice	1-3.OK	Good Choice
CaAl Hybrid	Good Choice	Good Choice	Good Choice	Good Choice	Good Choice	Good Choice	Good Choice	NO	Good Choice	1.GoodChoice 2.Good choice 3. NO	Good Choice

6.5 A clinical guide to selecting a permanent cement

Fig. 6.3 presents an overview of generic cements recommended for cementation of various clinical appliances that require permanent cementation. This figure has evolved and has been updated over a span of about 15 years and is expected to undergo modifications over time when new cements are introduced.

This guide is meant to help the practitioner with the selection of a luting agent. It refers to a generic choice, which then can be used by consulting Table 6.1 for a final choice of material. The guide is by no means intended to present a definitive, inflexible choice, but is intended to guide the practitioner towards the most likely appropriate material.

6.6 Properties of permanent luting agents

A list of 16 properties for generically listed cements can be seen in Tables 6.2 and 6.3.

Figure 6.3 Clinical indications for the use of luting agents. 1. Pameijer, C.H., Stanley, H.R., Ecker, G., 1988. Biocompatibility of glass ionomer luting agent in primates, Part I. Am. J. Dent. 1 (2), 71–76. 2. Pameijer, C.H., Stanley, H.R., 1991. Biocompatibility of glass ionomer luting agent, Part II, Crown Cementation. Am. J. Dent. 4, 134–142. 3. Pameijer, C.H., Stanley, H.R., 1992. Pulp reactions to resin cements. Am. J. Dent. 5, 81–87. 4. Pameijer, C.H., Nilner, K., 1994. Long term clinical evaluation of three luting agents. Swedish Dent. J. 18 (1–2), 59–67. 5. Pameijer, C.H., Jefferies S.R., 1996. Retentive properties and film thickness of 18 luting agents and luting systems. Gen. Dent. 44, 524–530. 6. Duncan, J., Pameijer, C.H., 1998. Retention of parallel-sided titanium posts with six luting agents, an in vitro study. J. Prosthet. Dent. 80, 423–428. 7. Lööf, J., Svahn, F., Jamar, T., Engqvist, H., Pameijer, C.H., 2007. A comparative study of the bioactivity of three dental materials. Dent. Mat. 24, 653–659. 8. Pameijer, C.H., Jefferies S.R., Lööf J., Hermansson L., 2008. A comparative crown retention test using XeraCem. J. Dent. Res. 87, Abstr #3099. 9. Jefferies S., Pameijer C.H., Appleby, D., Boston, D., Glantz P.-O., 2009 One year clinical performance and post-operative sensitivity of a bioactive dental luting cement—a prospective clinical pilot study. Swedish Dent. J. 33, 192–199. 10. Jefferies, S.R., Pameijer, C.H., Appleby, D., Boston, D., Lööf, J., Glantz, P.-O., 2013. Ceramir C&B, a bioactive dental luting cement—its retentive properties and three year clinical findings. Compend. Contin. Edu. Dent. 34(1), 2–9.

Table 6.2 **Comparison of parameters of various generic cements**

Cement	Universal	Retention	Biocompatibility	Sensitivity	Integration	Self-Etch	Self-Seal	Bioactive	Oxygen-inhibited layer
ZincPhosph	No	Low/Med	*	Yes	No	No	No	No	No
Polycarb	No	Low	****	No	No	No	No	No	No
Glass Ion	No	Medium	***	Yes	No	No	No	No	No
Resin	No	Medium	***	No	No	No	No	No	Yes
RMGI	Yes	Med/high	***	?	No	No	No	No	Yes
Self-Etch	Yes	High	****	?	?	Yes	No	No	Yes
Hybrid CaAl/GI	Yes	High	*****	No	Yes	Yes	Yes	Yes	No

RMGI, resin-modified glass ionomer.

Table 6.3 Comparison of additional parameters of the various generic cements

Cement	Nano-crystals	Hydroxy-apatite	Hydrolysis	Water sorption	Resin-based	Minerali-zing	*F*-release
ZincPhosph	No	No	No	No	No	No	No
Polycarb	No	No	No	No	No	No	No
Glass Ion	No	No	No	No	No	Yes	Yes
Resin	No	No	Yes	No	Yes	No	Yes
RMGI	No	No	Yes	Yes	Yes	No	Yes
Self-Etch	No	No	Yes	Yes	Yes	No	Yes
Hybrid CaAl/GI	Yes	Yes	No	No	No	Yes	Yes*

*Low.

6.7 Summary

Dramatic changes in chemistry and physical properties of cements during the last 100+ years have resulted in a market that offers so many choices that it comes as no surprise that many practitioners are confused when they have to determine what is best for the patient, given the clinical circumstances. This chapter's objectives were to comprehensively describe dental cements with an emphasis on biocompatibility. It is hoped that with the help of Fig. 6.3, the practitioner is guided towards an appropriate choice, rather than making arbitrary decisions, or decisions based on (often outdated) daily routine dentistry.

References

Al-Harbi, F.A., Ayad, N.M., Khan, Z.A., Mahrous, A.A., Morgano, S.M., 2015. In vitro shear bond strength of Y-TZP ceramics to different core materials with the use of three primer/resin cement systems. J. Prosthet. Dent. Sep 24. pii: S0022-3913(15)00399-6. http://dx.doi.org/10.1016/j.prosdent.2015.07.002. [Epub ahead of print].

Altintas, S.H., Tak, O., Secilmis, A., Usumez, A., 2011. Effect of provisional cements on shear bond strength of porcelain laminate veneers. Europ. J. Dent. 5, 373–379.

Anusavice, K.J., 1991. Phillips' Science of Dental Materials, 10th edition W.B. Saunders, Philadelphia, PA.

Bagis, B., Bagis, Y.H., Hasanreisoğlu, U., 2011. Bonding effectiveness of a self-adhesive Resin-based luting cement to dentin after provisional cement contamination. J. Adhes. Dent. 13, 543–550.

Blatz, M.B., Mante, F.K., Saleh, N., Atlas, A.M., Mannan, S., Ozer, F., 2013. Postoperative tooth sensitivity with a new self-adhesive resin cement—a randomized clinical trial. Clin. Oral Investig. 17, 793–798.

Bunek, S.S., Powers, J.M., 2012. Crown and bridge cements: clinical applications. Dent. Today 31 (42), 44–45.

Felton, D.A., Kanoy, B.E., White, J.T., 1987. Effect of cavity varnish on retention of cemented cast crowns. J. Prosthet. Dent. 57, 411–416.

Frankenberger, R., Hartmann, V.E., Krech, M., Krämer, N., Reich, S., Braun, A., et al., 2015. Adhesive luting of new CAD/CAM materials. Int. J. Comput. Dent. 18, 9–20.
Godoy-Bezerra, J., Vieira, S., Oliveira, J.H., Lara, F., 2006. Shear bond strength of resin-modified glass ionomer cement with saliva present and different enamel pretreatments. Angle Orthod. 76 (3), 470–474.
Goldberg, M., 2008. In vitro and in vivo studies on the toxicity of dental resin components: a review. Clin. Oral Investig. 12 (1), 1–8.
Greenland, L., 1974. The addition of fluoride to polycarboxylate cement. Univ. Toronto Undergrad. Dent. J. 10, 12–13.
Jefferies, S., Pameijer, C.H., Appleby, D., Boston, D., Glantz, P.-O., 2009. One year clinical performance and post-operative sensitivity of a bioactive dental luting cement—a prospective clinical pilot study. Swed. Dent. J. 33, 193–199.
Jefferies, S.R., Pameijer, C.H., Appleby, D., Boston, D., Lööf, J., Glantz, P.-O., 2013. Ceramir C&B, A bioactive dental luting cement—its retentive properties and three year clinical findings. Compend. Contin. Educ. Dent. 34, 2–9.
Jefferies, S.R., Fuller, A.E., Boston, D.W., 2015. Preliminary evidence that bioactive cements occlude artificial marginal gaps. J. Esthet. Restor. Dent. 27, 155–166.
Liu, Q., Meng, X., Yoshida, K., Luo, X., 2011. Bond degradation behavior of self-adhesive cement and conventional resin cements bonded to silanized ceramic. J. Prosthet. Dent. 105, 177–184.
Lööf, J., Svahn, F., Jarmar, T., Engqvist, H., Pameijer, C.H., 2008. A comparative study of the bioactivity of three materials for dental applications. Dent. Mat. 24, 653–659.
Martins, A.R., Gotti, V.B., Shimano, M.M., Borges, G.A., Gonçalves Lde, S., 2015. Improving adhesion between luting cement and zirconia-based ceramic with an alternative surface treatment. Braz. Oral. Res. 29, 54.
Nicholson, J.,W., Czarnecka, B., 2008. The biocompatibility of resin-modified glass-ionomer cements for dentistry. Dent. Mat. 24, 1702–1708.
Pameijer, C.H., 1992. On the clinical performance of a glass ionomer cement. biological, technological and clinical assessment of luting cements. Swed. Dent. J. Suppl. 80, 1–116.
Pameijer, C.H., Stanley, H.R., 1988. Biocompatibility of a glass ionomer luting agent in primates. Part I. Am. J. Dent. 1, 71–76.
Pameijer, C.H., Wendt Jr, S.L., 1995. Microleakage of various surface-seal materials. Am. Dent. J. 8, 43–46.
Pameijer, C.,H., Stanley, H.R., Ecker, G., 1991. Biocompatibility of a glass ionomer luting agent. 2. Crown cementation. Am. J. Dent. 4, 134–141.
Pashley, D.H., Tay, F.R., Yiu, C., et al., 2004. Collagen degradation by host-derived enzymes during aging. J. Dent. Res. 83, 216–221.
Ribeiro, J.C.V., Coelho, P.G., Janal, M.N., Silva, N.R.F.A., Monteiro, A.J., Fernandes, C.A.O., 2011. The influence of temporary cements on dental adhesive systems for luting cementation. J. Dent. 39, 255–262.
Ricci, H.A., Sanabe, M.E., de Souza Costa, C.A., Pashley, D.H., Hebling, J., 2010. Chlorhexidine increases the longevity of in vivo resin-dentin bonds. Eur. J. Oral Sci. 118, 411–416. Erratum in: Eur. J Oral Sci. 2010. 118,535.
Silva, J.P., Queiroz, D.M., Azevedo, L.H., Leal, L.C., Rodrigues, J.L., Lima, A.F., et al., 2011. Effect of eugenol exposure time and post-removal delay on the bond strength of a self-etching adhesive to dentin. Oper. Dent. 36, 66–71.
Smith, D.C., 1971. A review of the zinc polycarboxylate cements. J. Can. Dent. Assoc. 37, 22–29.
Stanley, H.R., 1981. Human Pulp Response to Restorative Procedures. Storter Printing, Gainesville, FL.
Wilson, A.D., Kent, B.E., 1972. A new translucent cement for dentistry. The glass ionomer cement. Br. Dent. J. 15, 133–135.

Biocompatibility of dental amalgams

7

Y. Uçar[1] *and W. Brantley*[2]
[1]Cukurova University, Balcali, Adana, Turkey; [2]The Ohio State University, Columbus, OH, United States

Abstract

This chapter discusses the biocompatibility of dental amalgam, which remains controversial for this widely used restorative material. Information is presented on the description, manipulation, composition, structure, and properties of dental amalgam, and the clinical behavior of dental amalgam restorations. Articles on biocompatibility of dental amalgam restorations are reviewed, notably recent clinical studies. While studies indicate that properly placed restorations present no health hazards, further research is needed to ensure that released mercury does not cause adverse physiological changes. The chapter concludes with guidelines for manipulating dental amalgam to avoid biocompatibility concerns and the current state of research in this field.

Chapter Outline

Biocompatibility of Dental Biomaterials. DOI: http://dx.doi.org/10.1016/B978-0-08-100884-3.00007-2

7.1 General description, clinical uses and manipulation of dental amalgam

Dental amalgam is an alloy used as a filling (restorative) material for tooth cavities caused by either decay, trauma, or other factors, and is composed of mercury, silver, tin, and copper, along with other metallic elements added to improve physical and mechanical properties (ADA, 2011). Dental amalgam has been a dental restorative material for almost 200 years (Greener, 1979; Eggleston, 1989; George et al., 2009; Anusavice et al., 2012). There are many reasons for this extended time of clinical existence. Dental amalgam is prepared easily, and it is relatively inexpensive compared with most other restorative materials used in dental treatment. The longevity of dental amalgam restorations is high (Roulet, 1997). The manipulation of dental amalgam after placement in the prepared tooth cavity is easy. The material has low creep, high compressive strength, and high resistance to wear, and it experiences minimal dimensional change with time (George et al., 2009; ADA, 2011; Uçar and Brantley, 2011). There is no other dental material known for marginal-sealing capacity that occurs with time after the restoration is placed in the oral cavity, which results in low microleakage. This property is attributed to the corrosion products released from dental amalgam restorations (Swartz and Phillips, 1961; ADA, 2011; Anusavice et al., 2012). The clinical placement of a dental amalgam restoration is not as technique-sensitive to operating conditions, such as the presence of saliva in the oral environment, compared with most other restorative materials (only applicable to the widely used zinc-free products discussed later). However, dental amalgam is probably the most controversial dental material because of biocompatibility concerns related to its high mercury content. Approximately 50% (wt.) of dental amalgam is elemental mercury, and a low level of it is released as mercury vapor that can be inhaled (US FDA, 2015).

Dental amalgam must be placed in a correctly prepared tooth cavity. Since dental amalgam is not able to bond to the tooth structure, mechanical retention is critical. The cavity is prepared according to certain principles (Heymann et al., 2012) originally established by G.V. Black: (1) The cavity outline should be rounded rather than having sharp edges. (2) The cavity walls should be retentive by provision of undercuts. (3) The preparation should be as conservative as possible to protect the pulp and the remaining tooth structure. Nevertheless, the strength of the restoration should be considered as well. The structural strength preservation of both the tooth structure and the amalgam restoration is important. Otherwise, thin sections of dental amalgam can lead to weakened restoration. (4) The mesial outline should be parallel to the distal wall, while the buccal outline should be parallel to the lingual wall. (5) The pulpal floor should be flat in order to increase the strength of amalgam restoration. (6) The internal angles should be rounded to avoid stresses both on the tooth structure and the restoration.

Dental amalgam is indicated clinically for Black cavities I, II, and V, and prevention of caries, as discussed in textbooks on operative dentistry (Heymann et al., 2012). Black I cavities occur on the occlusal surfaces of premolar and molar teeth, and on the lingual surfaces of maxillary incisors. Black II cavities include the restoration of proximal surfaces of posterior teeth in addition to the occlusal surfaces. Black V cavities are involved on the cervical third of the vestibular teeth or the lingual surfaces of all teeth.

The contraindications for the clinical use of dental amalgam can be listed as teeth where (1) esthetics is a high priority for the patient, (2) extensive destruction has occurred, or (3) very small cavities need to be restored.

Although dental amalgam was originally prepared by mixing the alloy for dental amalgam powder and high-purity dental mercury by hand (mortar and pestle), using mechanical means (amalgamators) is the preferred method (Heymann et al., 2012). Contemporarily, dental amalgam is marketed in capsules prepared by the manufacturer, which are mixed using mechanical devices, and the process is called trituration. This mixing enables a workable mass to be achieved and removes oxides from the mixture. During trituration, the powder particles partially dissolve in mercury, and a much more homogenous mixture is achieved when mixed using amalgamators, with the least possible amount of mercury used.

Once the homogeneous mixture is prepared, the mixed dental amalgam is placed in the prepared cavity and packed using an amalgam condenser (Heymann et al., 2012). This process is repeated layer-by-layer until the cavity is completely filled. Using carving instruments, the restoration is shaped appropriately, and then finalized by burnishing, and later, polishing steps.

7.2 History of dental amalgams and evolution of products

The history of dental amalgams and the evolution of commercial products are succinctly presented in an excellent review article (Mahler, 1997). The rich tapestry of earlier metallurgical research on this remarkable material is summarized in another excellent research article (Johnson and Wilsdorf, 1972).

The compositions of the traditional low-copper dental amalgams date from the extensive research by G.V. Black near the end of the 19th century. Historically, the starting alloy particles (lathe-cut or filed from a cast ingot) to be mixed with mercury contained at least 65 wt.% silver, 29 wt.% tin, and less than 6 wt.% copper (refer to Section 7.3 for setting reaction of low copper amalgam). Subsequently, a new alloy for dental amalgam was developed serendipitously in the early 1960s with the goal of providing a dispersion-strengthened dental amalgam; this high-copper alloy contained a mixture of low-copper dental amalgam particles and particles having the silver–copper eutectic composition of approximately 72 wt.% Ag and 28 wt.% Cu (Innes and Youdelis, 1963). While the promise of greatly improved mechanical properties was not achieved, this new alloy (subsequently named Dispersalloy for the widespread commercial product) was found to yield restorations with superior corrosion resistance because of the absence of the γ_2 phase in the microstructure. Subsequently, another high-copper alloy for dental amalgam was introduced (Asgar, 1974) in which all particles had the same composition, and this alloy, which did not form the γ_2 phase, also had excellent clinical performance (refer to Section 7.3 for the setting reaction of high copper amalgam). Currently, there are a large numbers of commercial dental amalgam products that meet the standards (e.g., ANSI/ADA, 2003; IOS, 2004), and should produce clinically satisfactory restorations when properly manipulated and expertly placed in the prepared tooth. Particles of the alloy powder can be lathe-cut or spherical, and particle size distributions are carefully controlled by the manufacturers to enable optimum condensation with minimal porosity in the restoration. Products are provided in preproportioned capsules containing liquid mercury in one compartment and the alloy particles in the other compartment. The mercury-to-alloy ratio is dependent on the type of alloy and is carefully controlled by the manufacturer to control the working and setting times and to provide optimum mechanical properties.

7.3 Setting reactions, metallurgical phases, and properties for dental amalgams

The setting reactions, microstructural phases, and properties for the different types of dental amalgams are described in textbooks on dental materials (O'Brien, 2008; Anusavice et al., 2012; Powers and Sakaguchi, 2013). These three general aspects are interrelated in a frequently complicated manner and are important for the biocompatibility of dental amalgams. These important areas are summarized in this section, with historically important references provided.

The setting reaction when the low-copper, G.V. Black-type alloys for dental amalgam are mixed with high-purity dental mercury can be written as:

$$\gamma\ (\text{Alloy}) + \text{Hg} \rightarrow \gamma_1 + \gamma_2 + \text{Unreacted Alloy.}$$

This form of the reaction emphasizes that the starting alloy particles are incompletely consumed when the reaction is completed; this is the case for all dental amalgams.

The original Dispersalloy product and similar admixture high-copper dental amalgam products, which contain low-copper dental amalgam particles and particles having the Ag–Cu eutectic composition, undergo a slower two-stage setting reaction when mixed with mercury, and the eventual setting reaction can be written as:

$$\gamma\ (\text{Alloy}) + \text{Hg} \rightarrow \gamma_1 + \eta' + \text{Unreacted Alloy.}$$

The first stage is identical to that for the low-copper dental amalgams, and the second stage involves the subsequent disappearance of the γ_2 phase, with formation of the η' phase.

The high-copper dental amalgams containing single-composition particles of the alloy for dental amalgam should not form the corrosion-prone γ_2 phase when mixed with mercury, and the more rapid setting reaction can also be written as:

$$\gamma\ (\text{Alloy}) + \text{Hg} \rightarrow \gamma_1 + \eta' + \text{Unreacted Alloy.}$$

However, a limited amount of γ_2 was found in one high-copper single-composition dental amalgam product containing indium (Marshall and Marshall, 1981).

Detailed information about the compositions of phases in the microstructures of dental amalgams has been obtained by quantitative microprobe analyses (Mahler, 1988, 1997; Mahler and Adey, 1984, 1988; Mahler et al., 1975) and X-ray energy-dispersive spectroscopic analyses with the scanning electron microscope (SEM) (Marshall and Marshall, 1981).

The starting particles of the alloy for dental amalgam that are mixed with mercury have a multiphase composition, consisting of γ (Ag_3Sn), β (Ag_4Sn), and ε (Cu_3Sn). Manufacturers employ a proprietary heat treatment to reduce compositional inhomogeneity and internal stress for these particles, which enables control of working and setting times. The phases that form during the setting reactions largely have the compositions of Ag_2Hg_3 (γ_1), Sn_8Hg (γ_2) and Cu_6Sn_5 (η'); however, these phases also contain small amounts of other elements, notably Sn in γ_1.

The γ_1 matrix in both low-copper and high-copper dental amalgams forms fine grains that are revealed by chemical etching of polished surfaces. The secondary γ_2 phase in low-copper dental amalgams, which undergoes corrosion, is interconnected in the microstructure (Jørgensen and Saito, 1970; Holland and Asgar, 1974), providing a pathway for surface corrosion to reach the interior of these restorations. Limited surface corrosion is beneficial for low-copper dental amalgam restorations, because the corrosion products inhibit marginal microleakage with time (margin-sealing). While the η' phase in high-copper dental amalgams undergoes corrosion, it is not interconnected in the microstructure, and beneficial corrosion processes that occur at the surface do not propagate into the interior. The η' phase in Dispersalloy-type high-copper dental amalgams forms, along with the γ_1 phase, in reaction rings at the peripheries of well-separated Ag–Cu eutectic composition particles. The η' phase exists as well-separated particles in the γ_1 matrix of the single-particle composition high-copper dental amalgams (Okabe et al., 1977; Mahler and Adey, 1984).

A delta (δ_2) phase has also been reported in dental amalgams from both differential scanning calorimetric and X-ray diffraction analyses (Sarkar et al., 1985; Sarker and Eyer, 1986; Söderholm, 1987). However, the existence of this phase in dental amalgams is controversial, and further research is needed to establish its presence definitively.

The multiphase microstructure of dental amalgams, also containing some porosity after condensation, imparts brittle character under normal rates of loading. Accordingly, the compressive strength and flexural strength are much greater than the tensile strength, since failure involves crack propagation. Values are provided in textbooks (O'Brien, 2008; Anusavice et al., 2012; Powers and Sakaguchi, 2013). The substantial differences in mechanical properties for the different loading modes are the basis of the manipulation procedures and cavity design principles for dental amalgam restorations.

Dental amalgam can also exhibit viscoelastic behavior (loading-rate dependence of mechanical properties). Creep under static loading (Mahler and Van Eysden, 1969) has been correlated with clinical marginal fracture of low-copper dental amalgam restorations (Mahler et al., 1986), and creep became an important property for laboratory evaluation in the dental amalgam standards. The current versions (ANSI/ADA, 2003; IOS, 2004) present the testing protocol.

A regression analysis for the in vitro creep of numerous dental amalgam products found that the relevant variables were volume percent of the η' phase, grain size of the γ_1 phase, volume percent of the γ and ε phases (in the unconsumed starting alloy particles), and the number of very small η' crystals per linear distance in high-magnification SEM micrographs (Mahler and Adey, 1991). This model was consistent with SEM examination of dental amalgams during creep, which revealed grain-boundary sliding in the γ_1 matrix. A much lower creep rate was observed for a γ_2–free high-copper amalgam than for a γ_2-containing low-copper amalgam (Okabe et al., 1983). This difference arises from the η' phase blocking the grain-boundary sliding of γ_1. An in vitro study found decreased creep in an aged low-copper dental amalgam from the formation of β_1 grains (Okabe et al., 1985).

7.4 Long-term clinical changes and failures of dental amalgam restorations

One long-term clinical change in dental amalgam restorations is corrosion, and corrosion products have been analyzed for clinically retrieved low-copper and high-copper dental amalgams, along with complementary in vitro studies (Marshall and Marshall, 1980, 1992; Marshall et al., 1982, 1987). The major corrosion products found in retrieved restorations with moderate clinical deterioration were tin oxides and tin hydroxychloride for both low-copper and high-copper amalgams.

A correlation was reported between in vitro corrosion of laboratory specimens measured by potentiodynamic cyclic polarization and in vivo marginal fracture for dental amalgam restorations reported from three independent research groups (Sarkar et al., 1982). However, there has been criticism that the data presented in this article do not support its conclusions (Mahler, 1983). An elegant discussion about the proper interpretation of the potentiodynamic polarization curves for dental amalgams has been presented (Olsson et al., 1997). Other studies have revealed how the corrosion resistance of dental amalgams can be altered by incorporating zinc (Sarkar and Park, 1988), palladium (Mahler et al., 1990) and indium (Johnson and Powell, 1992) in the starting alloy particles for dental amalgam, a strategy that has been employed by some manufacturers.

The long-term aging of dental amalgam also results in transformation of the γ_1 phase to the β_1 (Ag–Hg) phase, which has a lower mercury content. There is a release of mercury, which reacts with other phases, and the restorations do not contain free mercury. This transformation has been extensively studied in the laboratory (Johnson, 1967a,b; Espevik, 1977), and the presence of substantial β_1 phase has been observed in the microstructures of clinically retrieved low-copper and high-copper restorations (Boyer and Edie, 1990; Marshall et al., 1992).

It has been generally accepted that high-copper dental amalgam restorations perform better in clinical studies with lower incidence of marginal fracture and greater longevity, compared with low-copper dental amalgam restorations (Osborne et al., 1976; Wilson et al., 1996). However, this was not found in some long-term studies (Smales et al., 1991; Kreulen et al., 1998). A significant association was observed between clinical failure of dental amalgam restorations and surface tarnishing, but marginal fracture and marginal staining were not associated with three failure modes (Smales and Webster, 1993).

The clinical failure of dental amalgam restorations is still incompletely understood. Besides fracture at margins and in bulk restorations, along with creep and corrosion processes, which involve microstructural phases, laboratory evidence has been presented for combined creep and fatigue that might occur under cyclic functional forces in vivo (Williams and Hedge, 1985). It is plausible to expect that corrosion would also have some role in the cyclic fatigue process for clinical failure.

7.5 Older articles on health concerns with dental amalgam restorations

Health concerns about the use of mercury and dental amalgam restorations have persisted since this material was introduced in the 19th century (Greener, 1979). There was much research activity in the latter part of the 20th century, with now often-classic articles, that examined concerns for dentists and patients regarding dental amalgam restorations, and several important studies are summarized in this section.

In a comprehensive review article, Okabe (1987) pointed out that when liquid mercury does not contain an oxide film, it has a high vapor pressure and will evaporate at room temperature; moreover, the vapor pressure of mercury increases rapidly with temperature. It was emphasized that the high sensitivity of modern analytical equipment for mercury detection stimulated renewed public and scientific interest in the safety of dental amalgam restorations. Okabe (1987) reported laboratory data showing that the mercury vapor release from freshly prepared dental amalgam decreased rapidly after trituration and the completion of carving. Data obtained by Reynolds (1974), showed that the mercury evaporation rate from the γ_1 phase was over an order of magnitude greater than the evaporation rates from the β_1 and γ_2 phases; Reynolds (1974) found that the mercury evaporation rate from the γ_2 phase and a low-copper dental amalgam were similar and greater than the mercury evaporation rate from the Dispersalloy high-copper dental amalgam. Besides the long-term transformation of γ_1 to β_1, Okabe (1987) also noted that the γ_2 phase decomposes under clinical conditions. Uncertainty remains about the extent of further reaction of the mercury released from these transformations with microstructural phases, compared with evaporation from the dental restoration.

Reinhardt et al. (1983a) measured the level of mercury vapor expired by patients following removal of single dental amalgam restorations and found a small increase of about 10 minutes in duration that was avoidable with proper operative dentistry procedures (wet-field cutting, high-volume evacuation, and use of a rubber dam). A subsequent in vitro study (Reinhardt et al., 1983b) with a large number of dental amalgam specimens provided data supporting the in vivo study.

A theoretical article (Mackert, 1987) reviewed protocols for mercury vapor analyzers that had been employed by several research groups to measure levels in intraoral or expired air from patients with dental amalgam restorations. There was careful consideration of inhalation times and flow rates of air through the mouth during inhalation. It was concluded that a patient with a large number of occlusal restoration surfaces would receive a much smaller dose of mercury than the amount ingested from the normal intake of food, water and air (i.e., not occupationally exposed to mercury).

In a clinical study on patients with well-controlled diets, the estimated average daily dose of mercury vapor inhaled from dental amalgam restorations was much less than the threshold limit value (time-weighted average) of 0.05 mg/m^3 for airborne mercury set by the US government (National Institute for Occupational Safety and Health (NIOSH)) for an individual exposed for 8 hours per day for a 5-day working week (Berglund, 1990). For patients, there was very little effect on mercury vapor release with the number of restorations or the type of dental amalgam, and no effects were found for mercury levels in urine and saliva (Berglund, 1993). Further clinical study involving the removal of dental amalgam restorations from patients, with and without the use of rubber dams, revealed significant increases in the mercury levels in blood plasma and urine only for the patients without rubber dams; after 1 year, mercury levels in plasma and urine were substantially lower for the patients, compared with levels before removal of the restorations (Berglund and Molin, 1997).

In another investigation (Snapp et al., 1989), the mean baseline of total blood mercury was significantly correlated with the number of occlusal surfaces for adult subjects who had an average of 14 surfaces for dental amalgam restorations. After removal of these restorations, 9 of the 10 subjects exhibited a statistically significant decrease in blood mercury; it was also found that removal of the restorations caused an additional small exposure, evidenced by increased blood mercury levels, which disappeared within 3 days. The authors pointed out that evidence of mercury toxicity in the most sensitive adults appears at much greater Hg concentrations in blood, indicating that dental amalgam restorations do not appear to be a health hazard for patients.

To compare in vitro cytotoxicity, Wataha et al. (1994) placed extracts from Dispersalloy and a high-copper dental amalgam containing single-composition particles, obtained by incubating specimens in cell-culture medium for different times at 37°C, in contact with mouse fibroblasts for 24 hours and determined the succinic dehydrogenase activity of the cells. The high-copper dental amalgam containing single-composition particles exhibited no cytotoxicity compared with teflon controls. However, the Dispersalloy high-copper dental amalgam was severely cytotoxic initially when the release of Zn ions was greatest, but was less toxic between 48 and 72 hours as the Zn release decreased.

7.6 Recent articles demonstrating biocompatibility of dental amalgam restorations

There are many recently published papers that focus on the biocompatibility concerns for dental amalgam because of its high mercury content and the inhalation by patients of mercury vapor released from restorations. As explained previously, the mercury vapor concentration in the oral cavity is very low; moreover, the dental amalgam restorations are relatively small in size. Other forms of mercury that can be released from dental amalgam are of minimal importance.

7.6.1 In vitro studies

In vitro studies reside at the bottom of the evidence pyramid (Forrest, 2009). Nonetheless, they provide an important starting point to establish a platform for follow-up in vivo studies.

In vitro studies on the biocompatibility and toxicology of dental amalgam have been conducted in two different ways. Both rat and human cells have served as laboratory models.

Composite resins are advocated to patients as mercury-free alternatives to dental amalgam for restorations. Not only the absence of mercury release, but also the tooth-colored appearance of these polymeric materials, are presented as major benefits. In vitro studies have been conducted using human gingival fibroblasts to compare the cytotoxicity of resin-based materials with dental amalgam. Balto and Al-Nazhan (2003) evaluated the attachment of human periodontal ligament fibroblasts to three different root-end filling materials (gutta-percha, Super EBA and dental amalgam). The authors concluded that gutta-percha provided the best cell attachment and growth, followed by Super EBA, which was found to be better than dental amalgam. Although increased cell attachment is not the same as cytotoxicity, it gives an idea of whether the material surface is well tolerated by the cell. Reichl et al. evaluated both the cell death effect (Reichl et al., 2006a) and the cytotoxicity (Reichl et al., 2006b) of resin materials and dental amalgam at different concentrations over 48 hours; however, it was not clear how these concentrations related to the release that occurs from either composite or amalgam restorations in the mouth. Composite resin components were found to have lower toxicities than $HgCl_2$ or methyl mercury chloride proposed to represent dental amalgam (Reichl et al., 2006a). Their second study (Reichl et al., 2006b) reported the range of cytotoxicities for composite resin components, along with a time-dependent decrease in cytotoxicity for Hg^{2+}, which approached the toxicity level observed for *bis*-phenol-A-diglycidylmethacrylate (*bis*-GMA).

7.6.2 Studies on cadavers

Guzzi et al. (2006) evaluated mercury levels in autopsy tissues from 18 cadavers. Total mercury levels in brain, thyroid, and kidney samples were evaluated using atomic absorption spectroscopy. The group reported an increased amount of mercury in all types of tissues for an increasing number of dental amalgam restorations. Nevertheless, because of the small sample size and missing information about the intake of mercury from food (especially fish) or from occupational or environmental exposure, it was not possible to establish a definitive correlation between the mercury levels in autopsy tissues and the number of dental amalgam restorations. The total mercury levels in the brain were reported to be higher than the total mercury levels in the other autopsy tissues.

Another cadaver study, recently published by Ertaş et al. (2014), compared brain mercury levels in cadavers with (N = 10) and without (N = 22) dental amalgam restorations. The parietal lobes of the brains were analyzed using atomic absorption spectroscopy. Mercury was detected in 6 of the 10 cadavers with dental amalgam restorations, but was also detected in 8 of the 22 cadavers without dental amalgam restorations. The average mercury level in the brains of the dental amalgam group (0.97 ± 0.83) was slightly less than that for the dental amalgam-free group (1.06 ± 0.57).

7.6.3 In vivo studies

In addition to in vitro and cadaver studies, considerable research has been conducted in vivo to evaluate the correlation between the number of dental amalgam restorations and the mercury level in blood, serum, urine, hair, and saliva. Epidemiologic studies and clinical trials also are included in this group. There are only two published randomized, controlled clinical trials on dental amalgam (Children's Amalgam Trial), which were conducted in New England (Bellinger et al., 2007) and Portugal (DeRouen et al., 2006), and over 500 children were included in each study. The New England children were followed for 5 years, whereas the children in the other study were followed for 7 years. Neither of the studies found a difference in neurobehavioral outcomes between the children groups having and not having dental amalgam restorations. However, a statistically significant increase in urinary mercury levels was observed in the dental amalgam groups for both trials.

Five years after the Portugal Clinical Trial by DeRouen et al. (2006), Geier et al. (2011) reanalyzed the same data, employing a different calculation method and statistical analysis. The time that dental amalgam restorations survived in the mouth and the individual exposure scores were also taken into consideration. The children examined were from Lisbon, Portugal, and were 8–12 years old at the inception of the parent study. However, in contrast to the parent study, children with preexisting neurological or developmental disabilities were excluded from the data analysis reported in the second study. A total of 462 children were reevaluated in this new study. In addition to the neurobehavioral and neurological evaluation, renal function, urinary Hg, and urinary porphyrin levels were also assessed in the new study. Furthermore, information was collected about the composition, number, size, and positioning of dental restorations in each child's mouth. Unlike the parent DeRouen et al. (2006) study, Geier et al. (2011) found statistically significant differences between the urine mercury levels and dental amalgam exposure in a dose-dependent manner, and emphasized that a follow-up period of decades would be advisable to determine accurately the long-term pathological adverse effects of dental amalgam. Geier et al. (2011) also pointed out the strengths of the parent study and the limitations of their study.

Very recently, this group published another study (Geier et al., 2013) on the relationship between mercury exposure from dental amalgam restorations and kidney integrity biomarkers. This article also presented a reanalysis of the parent study by DeRouen et al. (2006). Similar to their previous study, the Geier et al. (2013) publication used a different statistical model to evaluate dose-dependent correlation between the cumulative exposure to mercury from dental amalgam restorations and urinary levels of renal biomarkers. While a statistically significant correlation was initially found, after some statistical adjustments, the relationship between mercury level and urinary renal biomarkers was no longer significant. Nevertheless, this group concluded that their results suggested a contribution of mercury from dental amalgam restorations to ongoing kidney damage in a dose-dependent manner. However, future studies are required to determine whether mercury exposure from dental amalgam restorations significantly contributes to medically diagnosed kidney disease.

There is a common concern about adverse reactions from not only dental amalgam but also all other restorative dental materials. A national survey on adverse reactions to dental materials in the United Kingdom was reported by Scott et al. (2004). The highest proportion of patient-related adverse reactions were due to dental alloys ($N =$ 175), and 124 of these were oral lichenoid reactions that were associated with dental amalgam. Although the number of dental amalgam restorations placed per year is decreasing, dental amalgam is still the most placed dental material because of its long life-span, which can be up to 20 years (US FDA, 2015). Therefore, it is not surprising that dental amalgam is the most reported material for causing adverse reactions by patients. The ratio between the number of adverse reactions by patients and the total number of the current restorations in the oral cavities of the patient population should be considered.

Another comprehensive clinical study was conducted on Belgian children and their mothers (Pirard et al., 2014). The results confirmed that consumption of seafood was the most important determinant for the increase of mercury content in the hair. However, the presence of dental amalgam restorations was the second-highest determinant of hair mercury. Even the increased mercury levels, resulting from fish consumption, were much lower than the accepted level (7 μg/g) that does not cause health hazards for patients (US FDA, 2015).

Mercury levels in urine were evaluated in Spanish adults (Castaño et al., 2012) and higher mercury levels were found in urine for participants with dental amalgam restorations, although there was no evaluation of the effect of fish or seafood consumption. Moreover, there was no discussion about whether the increased mercury level in the dental amalgam patient group was clinically significant.

The effect of acute exposure to mercury from dental amalgam has been evaluated (Sandborgh-Englund et al., 2003) and indicated that mercury released from dental amalgam restorations does not increase the interlekin 6 (IL-6) and C-reactive protein levels, which shows that there is no sign of inflamation. Bárány et al. (2003) evaluated the effect of fish consumption and presence of dental amalgam restorations on mercury levels in the blood and serum of 245 adolescents, and reported that the mercury contribution from dental amalgam was much lower than that from fish and seafood.

Blood and urine mercury levels in adult patients having dental amalgam restorations were monitored in a randomized controlled trial (Halbach et al., 2008). The patients were monitored postremoval of the restorations for 180 days. The mean integrated daily dose (7.4 μg) received by the patients was much lower than the tolerable dose of 30 μg (US FDA, 2015).

Takahashi et al. (2001) evaluated both the release of mercury from dental amalgam in pregnant rats and the distribution of mercury in maternal and fetal tissues. Subsequently, Takahashi et al. (2003) investigated the placental transfer of mercury in pregnant rats. This group found that (1) the amounts of mercury in both the maternal and the fetal tissues of rats that had received dental amalgam restorations were higher compared with the controls that had not receive restorations, and (2) the mercury concentration in the fetal tissues was less than that in the maternal tissues. However, the question of whether the difference in mercury concentrations for the test and control groups had clinical significance was not examined. Investigation of the placental transfer of mercury in pregnant rats revealed that (1) the amount of mercury release was increased as the amalgam surface area increased, and (2) the mercury vapor released from dental amalgam restorations in pregnant rats was distributed to both maternal and fetal organs.

7.7 Guidelines related to biocompatibility for proper manipulation of dental amalgams

Mercury, even in small amounts. is a danger, not only for humans but also for the environment. Therefore, proper management of waste mercury is critical. Dental amalgam is also claimed to be one of the main sources of mercury pollution. The American Dental Association (ADA) reported that if properly managed, dental amalgam waste can be released into the environment. A document about "Best Management Practices for Amalgam Waste" (BMPs) has been developed by the ADA (http://www.ada.org) for handling dental amalgam waste, including using chair-side traps and vacuum collection, installing dental amalgam separators, and inspecting and cleaning traps, in addition to collecting and recycling scrap amalgam.

Mercury in dental amalgam contributes to the mercury contamination of wastewater. The US Environmental Protection Agency (EPA) estimated that in 2008 there were 122,000 dental offices that placed or removed dental amalgam restorations in the United States. The number of dental offices in developing countries that place dental amalgam restorations is probably also high. The US EPA estimates that approximately 3.7 tons of mercury are discharged annually to publicly owned treatment works (POTWs), and in 2003 dental offices were the source of 50% of all mercury pollution in US POTWs. The POTWs collect wastewater and transport it through a collection system to a treatment plant where the harmful organisms and contaminants are removed from the sewage. The EPA website (http://www.epa.gov) provides more detailed information about POTWs.

The US EPA notes that approximately 40% of the mercury in US wastewater comes from dental offices. Therefore, proper manipulation of dental amalgam is critical. The EPA stresses the importance of several precautions: (1) amalgam waste cannot be placed with regular garbage or with infectious waste; (2) chair-side traps or vacuum pump filters containing dental amalgam must not be rinsed over drains or sinks; (3) empty dental amalgam capsules must not be disposed with infectious waste or municipal waste that is incinerated; (4) amalgam waste must never be flushed down the drain. There are amalgam-recycling companies that collect waste dental amalgam from dental clinics. Waste dental amalgam is collected and carried in specially designed and manufactured sealed containers.

Contamination with bacterial aerosols having particle sizes from 5 to 50 μm is a major concern for dental clinics (Miller and Micik, 1978). Bio-aerosols are generated during dental procedures such as tooth cavity preparation, caries excavation, and cleaning or polishing teeth, and they remain airborne for several seconds. Aerosols created during caries excavation can contain *Streptococci mutans* and *sanguis* (Earnest and Loesche, 1991). Therefore, ventilation of operating rooms in dental clinics is critically important. The ventilation system should have highly efficient filters, and it is critical to have a negative pressure in the dental operatory compared to the other rooms in the office suite. Unfortunately, there is not any standard for ventilation of dental offices, and this is a highly important matter to be addressed by appropriate governmental agencies in countries where dental amalgam restorations are being placed in patients.

7.8 Current status of research on biocompatibility of dental amalgam restorations

High levels of mercury vapor exposure are associated with adverse effects in the brain and the kidneys. However, mercury released from dental amalgam restorations has been shown to be much lower than the mercury intake from other sources such as seafood, water, and industry.

The US FDA (2015) declares that dental amalgam is safe for use as a restorative material for adults and children aged at least 6 years. The amount of mercury measured in blood, plasma, saliva, breast milk, hair, brain, and liver is below the levels that cause adverse health effects. The US FDA has pointed out the limited clinical information available about potential effects of dental amalgam restorations on pregnant women, fetal tissues, and children below 6 years old. Although very rare, the US FDA reports that there are people who are sensitive to dental amalgam and, after dental restoration with this material, can have allergic reactions. The Life Sciences Research Office of the US FDA has conducted detailed research on dental amalgam and found insufficient evidence to conclude that this material causes health problems.

References

American Dental Association (ADA) Council on Scientific Affairs, 2011. Statement on dental amalgam. Available from: http://www.ada.org [Accessed 19 January 2015].

American National Standards Institute/American Dental Association (ANSI/ADA) Standard No. 1, 2003. Alloy for Dental Amalgam. American Dental Association, Chicago, IL.

Anusavice, K.J., Shen, C., Rawls, H.R., 2012. Phillips' Science of Dental Materials, 12th ed. Elsevier/Saunders, St. Louis, MO.

Asgar, K., 1974. Amalgam alloy with a single composition behavior similar to Dispersalloy (abstract). IADR Progr & Abstr 53, 60.

Balto, H., Al-Nazhan, S., 2003. Attachment of human periodontal ligament fibroblasts to 3 different root-end filling materials: scanning electron microscope observation. Oral Surg. Oral Med. Oral Pathol. Oral Radiol. Endod. 95, 222–227.

Bárány, E., Bergdahl, I.A., Bratteby, L.E., Lundh, T., Samuelson, G., Skerfving, S., et al., 2003. Mercury and selenium in whole blood and serum in relation to fish consumption and amalgam fillings in adolescents. J. Trace Elem. Med. Biol. 17, 165–170.

Bellinger, D.C., Daniel, D., Trachtenberg, F., Tavares, M., McKinlay, S., 2007. Dental amalgam restorations and children's neuropsychological function: the New England Children's Amalgam Trial. Environ. Health Perspect. 115, 440–446.

Berglund, A., 1990. Estimation by a 24-hour study of the daily dose of intra-oral mercury vapor inhaled after release from dental amalgam. J. Dent. Res. 69, 1646–1651.

Berglund, A., 1993. An in vitro and in vivo study of the release of mercury vapor from different types of amalgam alloys. J. Dent. Res. 72, 939–946.

Berglund, A., Molin, M., 1997. Mercury levels in plasma and urine after removal of all amalgam restorations: the effect of using rubber dams. Dent. Mater. 13, 297–304.

Boyer, D.B., Edie, J.W., 1990. Composition of clinically aged amalgam restorations. Dent. Mater. 6, 146–150.

Castaño, A., Sánchez-Rodríguez, J.E., Cañas, A., Esteban, M., Navarro, C., Rodríguez-García, A.C., et al., 2012. Mercury, lead and cadmium levels in the urine of 170 Spanish adults: a pilot human biomonitoring study. Int. J. Hyg. Environ. Health 215, 191–195.

DeRouen, T.A., Martin, M.D., Leroux, B.G., Townes, B.D., Woods, J.S., Leitão, J., et al., 2006. Neurobehavioral effects of dental amalgam in children: a randomized clinical trial. JAMA 19, 1784–1792.

Earnest, R., Loesche, W., 1991. Bacteria in dental aerosols. J. Am. Dent. Assoc. 122, 55–57.

Eggleston, D.W., 1989. Dental amalgam: a review of the literature. Compendium 10, 500–505.

Ertaş, E., Aksoy, A., Turla, A., Karaarslan, E., Karaarslan, B., Aydın, A., et al., 2014. Human brain mercury levels related to exposure to amalgam fillings. Hum. Exp. Toxicol. 33, 873–877.

Espevik, S., 1977. Creep and phase transformation in dental amalgam. J. Dent. Res. 56, 36–39.

Forrest, J.L., 2009. Introduction to the basics of evidence-based dentistry: concepts and skills. J. Evid. Based Dent. Pract. 9, 108–112.

Geier, D.A., Carmody, T., Kern, J.K., King, P.G., Geier, M.R., 2011. A significant relationship between mercury exposure from dental amalgams and urinary porphyrins: a further assessment of the Casa Pia children's dental amalgam trial. Biometals 24, 215–224.

Geier, D.A., Carmody, T., Kern, J.K., King, P.G., Geier, M.R., 2013. A significant dose-dependent relationship between mercury exposure from dental amalgams and urinary mercury levels: a further assessment of the Casa Pia Children's Dental Amalgam Trial. Hum. Exp. Toxicol. 31, 11–17.

George, G.N., Singh, S.P., Hoover, J., Pickering, I.J., 2009. The chemical forms of mercury in aged and fresh dental amalgam surfaces. Chem. Res. Toxicol. 22, 1761–1764.

Greener, E.H., 1979. Amalgam—yesterday, today, and tomorrow. Oper. Dent. 4, 24–35.

Guzzi, G., Grandi, M., Cattaneo, C., Calza, S., Minoia, C., Ronchi, A., et al., 2006. Dental amalgam and mercury levels in autopsy tissues: food for thought. Am. J. Forensic Med. Pathol. 27, 42–45.

Halbach, S., Vogt, S., Köhler, W., Felgenhauer, N., Welzl, G., Kremers, L., et al., 2008. Blood and urine mercury levels in adult amalgam patients of a randomized controlled trial: interaction of Hg species in erythrocytes. Environ. Res. 107, 69–78.

Heymann, H.O., Swift Jr., E.J., Ritter, A.V., 2012. Sturdevant's Art and Science of Operative Dentistry, 6th ed. Elsevier/Mosby, St. Louis, MO.

Holland, G.A., Asgar, K., 1974. Some effects on the phases of amalgam induced by corrosion. J. Dent. Res. 53, 1245–1254.

Innes, D.B.K., Youdelis, W.V., 1963. Dispersion strengthened amalgams. J. Can. Dent. Assoc. 29, 587–593.

International Organization for Standardization, 2004. ISO 24234: Dentistry—Mercury and alloys for dental amalgam. Geneva, Switzerland.

Johnson Jr., L.B., 1967a. X-ray diffraction evidence for the presence of β (Ag-Hg) in dental amalgam. J. Biomed. Mater. Res. 1, 285–297.

Johnson Jr., L.B., 1967b. Confirmation of the presence of β (Ag-Hg) in dental amalgam. J. Biomed. Mater. Res. 1, 415–425.

Johnson, Jr., L.B., Wilsdorf, H.G.F., 1972. Basic metallurgy of dental amalgam. National Bureau of Standards Special Publication 354, 43–59.

Johnson, G.H., Powell, L.V., 1992. Effect of admixed indium on properties of a dispersed-phase high-copper dental amalgam. Dent Mater 8, 366–369.

Jørgensen, K.D., Saito, T., 1970. Structure and corrosion of dental amalgams. Acta Odontol. Scand. 28, 129–142.

Kreulen, C.M., Tobi, H., Gruythuysen, R.J.M., van Amerongen, W.E., Borgmeijer, P.J., 1998. Replacement risk of amalgam treatment modalities: 15-year results. J. Dent. 26, 627–632.

Mackert Jr., J.R., 1987. Factors affecting estimation of dental amalgam mercury exposure from measurements of mercury vapor levels in intra-oral and expired air. J. Dent. Res. 66, 1775–1780.

Mahler, D.B., 1983. Letter to the editor. J. Dent. Res. 62, 841.

Mahler, D.B., 1988. Research on dental amalgam: 1982–1986. Adv. Dent. Res. 2, 71–82.

Mahler, D.B., 1997. The high-copper dental amalgam alloys. J. Dent. Res. 76, 537–541.

Mahler, D.B., Adey, J.D., 1984. Microprobe analysis of three high-copper amalgams. J. Dent. Res. 63, 921–925.

Mahler, D.B., Adey, J.D., 1988. Sn in the Ag-Hg phase of dental amalgam. J. Dent. Res. 67, 1275–1277.

Mahler, D.B., Adey, J.D., 1991. Factors influencing the creep of dental amalgam. J. Dent. Res. 70, 1394–1400.

Mahler, D.B., Van Eysden, J., 1969. Dynamic creep of dental amalgam. J. Dent. Res. 48, 501–508.

Mahler, D.B., Adey, J.D., Van Eysden, J., 1975. Quantitative microprobe analysis of amalgam. J. Dent. Res. 54, 218–226.

Mahler, D.B., Engle, J.H., Adey, J.D., 1990. Effect of Pd on the clinical performance of amalgam. J. Dent. Res. 69, 1759–1761.

Mahler, D.B., Engle, J.H., Bryant, R.W., 1986. Standardizing evaluations of the clinical marginal fracture of amalgam. J. Dent. Res. 65, 1108–1111.

Marshall Jr., G.W., Marshall, S.J., 1981. X-ray diffraction and SEM/EDS analyses of phases in new dental amalgams. J. Oral. Rehabil. 8, 43–53.

Marshall Jr., G.W., Marshall, S.J., Letzel, H., Vrijhoef, M.M.A., 1987. Microstructures of Cu-rich amalgam restorations with moderate clinical deterioration. Dent. Mater. 3, 135–143.

Marshall, S.J., Marshall Jr., G.W., 1980. $Sn_4(OH)_6Cl_2$ and SnO corrosion products of amalgams. J. Dent. Res. 59, 820–823.

Marshall, S.J., Marshall Jr., G.W., 1992. Dental amalgam: the materials. Adv. Dent. Res. 6, 94–99.

Marshall, S.J., Lin, J.H., Marshall Jr., G.W., 1982. Cu_2O and $CuCl_2{\cdot}3Cu(OH)_2$ corrosion products on copper rich dental amalgams. J. Biomed. Mater. Res. 16, 81–85.
Marshall, S.J., Marshall Jr., G.W., Letzel, H., 1992. Gamma-1 to beta-1 phase transformation in retrieved clinical amalgam restorations. Dent. Mater. 8, 162–166.
Miller, R.L., Micik, R.E., 1978. Air pollution and its control in the dental office. Dent. Clin. North Am. 22, 453–476.
O'Brien, W.J., 2008. Dental Materials and Their Selection, 4th ed. Quintessence, Chicago, IL.
Okabe, T., 1987. Mercury in the structure of dental amalgam. Dent. Mater. 3, 1–8.
Okabe, T., Butts, M.B., Mitchell, R.J., 1983. Changes in the microstructures of silver-tin and admixed high-copper amalgams during creep. J. Dent. Res. 62, 37–43.
Okabe, T., Mitchell, R., Butts, M.B., Bosley, J.R., Fairhurst, C.W., 1977. Analysis of Asgar-Mahler reaction zone in Dispersalloy amalgam by electron diffraction. J. Dent. Res. 56, 1037–1043.
Okabe, T., Mitchell, R.J., Butts, M.B., Galloway, S.S., Twiggs, W.S., 1985. Change in creep rate and microstructure in an aged, low-copper amalgam. J. Biomed. Mater. Res. 19, 727–746.
Olsson, S., Bergman, M., Marek, M., Berglund, A., 1997. Connections between polarization curves and log (a_i/a_{ref})-pe diagram. J. Dent. Res. 76, 1869–1878.
Osborne, J.W., Phillips, R.W., Gale, E.N., Binon, P.P., 1976. Three-year clinical comparison of three amalgam alloy types emphasizing an appraisal of the evaluation methods used. J. Am. Dent. Assoc. 93, 784–789.
Pirard, C., Koppen, G., De Cremer, K., Van Overmeire, I., Govarts, E., Dewolf, M.C., et al., 2014. Hair mercury and urinary cadmium levels in Belgian children and their mothers within the framework of the COPHES/DEMOCOPHES projects. Sci. Total Environ. 15, 730–740.
Powers, J.M., Sakaguchi, R.L., 2013. Craig's Restorative Dental Materials, 13th ed. Elsevier/Mosby, St. Louis, MO.
Reichl, F.X., Esters, M., Simon, S., Seiss, M., Kehe, K., Kleinsasser, N., et al., 2006a. Cell death effects of resin-based dental material compounds and mercurials in human gingival fibroblasts. Arch. Toxicol. 80, 370–377.
Reichl, F.X., Simon, S., Esters, M., Seiss, M., Kehe, K., Kleinsasser, N., et al., 2006b. Cytotoxicity of dental composite (co)monomers and the amalgam component Hg^{2+} in human gingival fibroblasts. Arch. Toxicol. 80, 465–472.
Reinhardt, J.W., Boyer, D.B., Svare, C.W., Frank, C.W., Cox, R.D., Gay, D.D., 1983a. Exhaled mercury following removal and insertion of amalgam restorations. J. Prosthet. Dent. 49, 652–656.
Reinhardt, J.W., Chan, K.C., Schulein, T.M., 1983b. Mercury vaporization during amalgam removal. J. Prosthet. Dent. 50, 62–64.
Reynolds Jr., C.L., 1974. Determination of mercury vapor pressure over amalgams from weight loss data. J. Biomed. Mater. Res. 8, 369–373.
Roulet, J.F., 1997. Benefits and disadvantages of tooth-coloured alternatives to amalgam. J. Dent. 25, 459–473.
Sandborgh-Englund, G., Geijersstam, E., Loftenius, A., 2003. Acute exposure to mercury from dental amalgam does not affect the levels of C-reactive protein or interleukin-6 in peripheral blood. J. Toxicol. Environ. Health A 66, 495–499.
Sarkar, N.K., Eyer, C.S., 1986. Solid solubility of tin in silver-mercury γ_1 in dental amalgams. J. Oral Rehabil. 13, 559–566.
Sarkar, N.K., Park, J.-R., 1988. Mechanism of improved corrosion resistance of Zn-containing dental amalgams. J. Dent. Res. 67, 1312–1315.

Sarkar, N.K., Eyer, C.S., Koger, S., 1985. Detection of new phases in dental amalgams using DSC. Am. Lab. 17, 24–27.

Sarkar, N.K., Osborne, J.W., Leinfelder, K.F., 1982. *In vitro* corrosion and *in vivo* marginal fracture of dental amalgams. J. Dent. Res. 61, 1262–1268.

Scott, A., Egner, W., Gawkrodger, D.J., Hatton, P.V., Sherriff, M., van Noort, R., et al., 2004. The national survey of adverse reactions to dental materials in the UK: a preliminary study by the UK Adverse Reactions Reporting Project. Br. Dent. J. 24, 471–477.

Smales, R.J., Webster, D.A., 1993. Restoration deterioration related to later failure. Oper. Dent. 18, 130–137.

Smales, R.J., Webster, D.A., Leppard, P.I., 1991. Survival predictions of amalgam restorations. J. Dent. 19, 272–277.

Snapp, K.R., Boyer, D.B., Peterson, L.C., Svare, C.W., 1989. The contribution of dental amalgam to mercury in blood. J. Dent. Res. 68, 780–785.

Söderholm, K.-J.M., 1987. An x-ray diffractometric investigation of the Sn-Hg binary system within the 0-40% Hg interval. J. Dent. Res. 66, 712–715.

Swartz, M.L., Phillips, R.W., 1961. In vitro studies on the marginal leakage of restorative materials. J. Am. Dent. Assoc. 62, 141–151.

Takahashi, Y., Tsuruta, S., Arimoto, M., Tanaka, H., Yoshida, M., 2003. Placental transfer of mercury in pregnant rats which received dental amalgam restorations. Toxicology 185, 23–33.

Takahashi, Y., Tsuruta, S., Hasegawa, J., Kameyama, Y., Yoshida, M., 2001. Release of mercury from dental amalgam fillings in pregnant rats and distribution of mercury in maternal and fetal tissues. Toxicology 163, 115–126.

Uçar, Y., Brantley, W.A., 2011. Biocompatibility of dental amalgams. Int. J. Dent., 981595.

United States Food and Drug Administration (US FDA)—http://www.fda.gov [Accessed 19 January 2015].

Wataha, J.C., Nakajima, H., Hanks, C.T., Okabe, T., 1994. Correlation of cytotoxicity with elemental release from mercury- and gallium-based dental alloys *in vitro*. Dent. Mater. 10, 298–303.

Williams, P.T., Hedge, G.L., 1985. Creep-fatigue as a possible cause of dental amalgam margin failure. J. Dent. Res. 64, 470–475.

Wilson, N.H.F., Wastell, D.G., Norman, R.D., 1996. Five-year performance of high-copper content amalgam restorations in a multiclinical trial of a posterior composite. J. Dent. 24, 203–210.

Biocompatibility of oral care products

8

K. Moharamzadeh
University of Sheffield, Sheffield, United Kingdom

Abstract

This chapter will focus on the biocompatibility of oral care products including toothpastes, mouthwashes, tooth-whitening products, and denture care materials. Currently available biological test systems used for biocompatibility testing of oral care products are introduced. Various types of toothpastes and mouthwashes are discussed including their compositions, indications, current evidence on their clinical performance and biological concerns associated with the active ingredients as well as laboratory and clinical studies of their biocompatibility. Safety concerns regarding tooth-whitening products and current legislation and regulatory requirements are also included in this chapter. Biocompatibility issues concerning denture care products are discussed and, finally, important recommendations are suggested for dental care professionals regarding appropriate use and prescription of oral care products.

Chapter Outline

Biocompatibility of Dental Biomaterials. DOI: http://dx.doi.org/10.1016/B978-0-08-100884-3.00008-4

8.1 Introduction

Oral care products are defined as products used for care of the teeth and the mouth. Various products are available based on their special clinical indications including toothpastes, mouthwashes, tooth-whitening products, and denture care materials. Although these products have gone through standard safety evaluations prior to marketing, and have been approved by the regulatory bodies, local and systemic adverse reactions associated with different materials in each category have been reported.

There are fewer scientific studies addressing the biocompatibility issues associated with oral care products compared to those reporting on the efficacy of these products. A possible reason for the reduced amount of research in this area is the passive nature of the exposure of the oral tissues to these products. Since oral care products typically come into contact with oral tissues for a short period of time and are then rinsed away following exposure, there appears to be an assumption that any adverse effects on oral tissues are mitigated. In addition, there is a tendency for the manufacturers to sponsor more studies evaluating the positive effects of the oral care products in terms of efficacy and clinical performance compared with studies which would raise concerns on adverse reactions to these products. In this chapter, first we will introduce different biocompatibility test systems that are available for biological evaluation of oral care products, and then we will describe each category of product and discuss specific biocompatibility issues associated with different types of oral care products in more detail.

8.2 Biocompatibility test systems for the evaluation of oral care products

Biocompatibility is defined as "the ability of a material to function in a specific application in the presence of an appropriate host response" (Williams, 1987). Appropriate host response in dentistry in most cases means no adverse reaction of the living system to the tested materials. These reactions in patients can be divided into two main categories: (1) local adverse reactions, and (2) systemic adverse reactions. Different types of biocompatibility test systems have been developed to evaluate local and systemic biological effects of oral care products as demonstrated in Fig. 8.1.

Localized adverse effects of oral care products on oral mucosa can be investigated using two different types of biocompatibility test systems including in vitro and in vivo tests.

8.2.1 In vitro tests

In vitro tests are carried out outside of the body. Their objective is to simulate biological reactions to oral care products when they are placed on or into tissue of the body (Hanks et al., 1996). The in vitro tests are suitable for screening new oral care products compared with time-consuming and expensive animal studies. They are

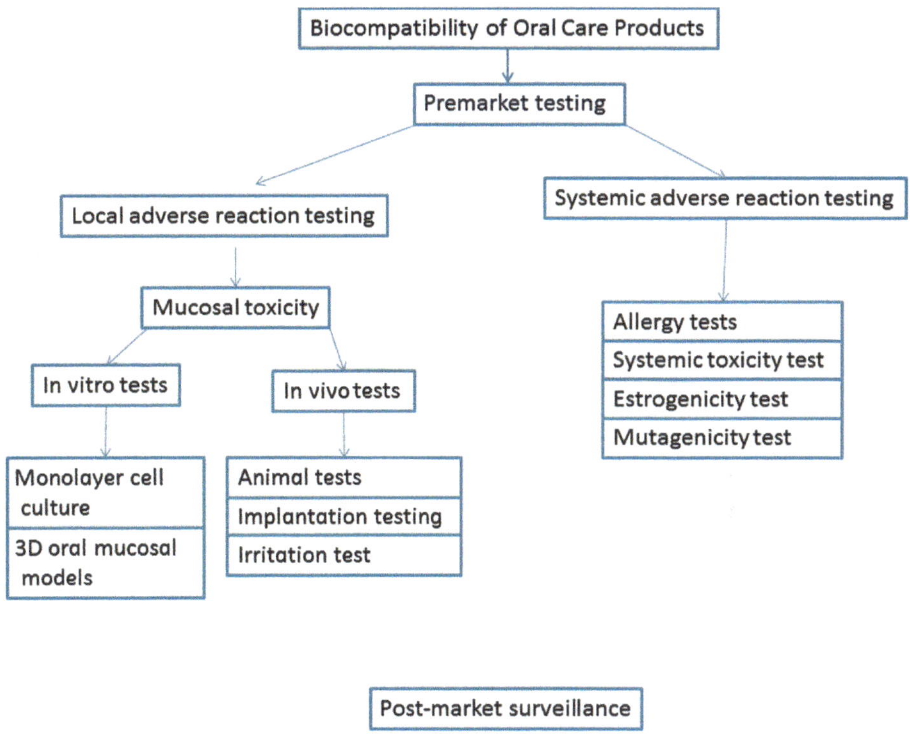

Figure 8.1 Biocompatibility tests relevant to oral care products.

more reproducible, controllable, relatively simple, and fast, with minimal ethical issues. The most commonly used biological system for in vitro evaluation of oral care products is monolayer cultures of human oral epithelial cells or fibroblasts. The main limitations of these systems are the lack of simulation of the in vivo situation and questionable clinical relevance. To obtain more accurate risk assessment and to reflect the clinical situation as closely as possible, three-dimensional tissue-engineered models of human oral mucosa have been developed recently for biological evaluation of dental materials and oral care products (Moharamzadeh et al., 2008a,b, 2009). These 3D tissue model systems have proved promising for the biological evaluation of dental materials and oral care products as they simulate the clinical situation better than monolayer cell culture systems and permit multiple-endpoint analysis of the response of human oral mucosa to tested materials. They may reduce or eliminate the need for animal tests and be more specific in terms of biological aspects to be assessed (Moharamzadeh et al., 2007, 2012).

8.2.2 In vivo tests

In vivo tests are carried out inside a living body. One of the common types of in vivo tests are animal implantation tests, in which the test material is implanted into the body of the animal to assess its localized adverse reactions. These tests permit examination of complex interactions between the living system and the test material, and therefore should be more clinically relevant than in vitro tests. Animal tests can be expensive, time-consuming, and sometimes it can be difficult to control specific variables. There are also ethical issues regarding the use of animals for research and questions in terms of the suitability of animals to represent the response of humans to the tested materials.

8.2.3 Systemic adverse reaction tests

Systemic adverse effects of oral care products have been investigated using mainly the following test systems: (1) systemic toxicity testing, and (2) allergic reaction testing. Systemic toxicity tests have been frequently used to investigate the characteristics and treatment of acute toxicity caused by ingested fluoride present in toothpastes and mouthwashes (Whitford, 2011). Allergic reactions such as anaphylaxis or contact dermatitis to various components of oral care products have also been reported (Lachapelle, 2014).

8.3 Biocompatibility of toothpastes

8.3.1 Composition of toothpastes

Toothpastes generally contain the following components:

- Water (20–40%)
- Abrasives (50%) including aluminum hydroxide, calcium hydrogen phosphates, calcium carbonate, silica and hydroxyapatite
- Fluoride (usually 1450 ppm) mainly in the form of sodium fluoride. Stannous fluoride and sodium monofluorophosphate have also been used
- Detergents, mainly sodium lauryl sulfate (SLS) with concentration ranges of 0.5–2%
- Antibacterial agents such as triclosan or zinc chloride
- Flavourants including spearmint, peppermint, and wintergreen
- Remineralizers in some toothpastes containing hydroxyapatite nanoparticles and calcium phosphate
- Humectants including glycerol, xylitol, sorbitol, polyethylene glycol, and propylene glycol
- Antisensitivity agents in sensitive toothpastes containing strontium chloride and potassium nitrate or arginine
- Anticalculus agents such as sodium polyphosphate or zinc citrate.

8.3.2 Biological studies

Safety concerns have been raised regarding several commonly used ingredients in toothpastes. Biological studies on toothpastes and reports of adverse reactions have been mainly associated with fluoride, SLS, and triclosan.

8.3.2.1 Fluoride

It has been shown that excessive fluoride concentrations (50–100 ppm) in drinking water can cause adverse effects such as neurotoxicity including effects on memory and learning (Chioca et al., 2008), as well as impaired neurodevelopment (Choi et al., 2012).

Ingesting large amounts of toothpastes containing fluoride can cause acute systemic toxicity which begins with gastric signs and symptoms, and can develop very rapidly. For example, ingestion of only 1.8 ounces of a standard fluoridated toothpaste (900–1100 mg/kg) by a 10-kg child delivers enough fluoride to reach the "probable toxic dose" (5 mg/kg body weight) (Whitford, 2011). Toothpastes with high fluoride content (above 1000 ppm) and pleasant flavours are more likely to reach a toxic dose if swallowed by children, especially when they are kept in nonsecure locations at home. Various factors including chemical composition, the age of the patient, and the time between the exposure and the treatment can affect the clinical presentation of an overexposure. It has been reported that young children aged below 6 years account for more than 80% of reports of suspected over-ingestion (Shulman and Wells, 1997). It is important to educate parents and childcare providers to handle fluoride-containing toothpastes carefully and to store them out of the reach of children to prevent the possibility of their ingestion (Whitford, 1987). Manufacturers should also be encouraged to use child-proof packaging for all fluoride-containing oral care home products.

Chronic exposure of young children to fluoride during tooth formation can also increase the risk of developing dental fluorosis (Denbesten and Li, 2011). Fluoride interferes with the tooth mineralization process through various mechanisms. Fluoride can either directly affect the ameloblasts or interact with the proteins and enzymes such as proteinase in the developing enamel matrix. A delay in enamel proteins (amelogenins) removal during the maturation stage can lead to formation of porous enamel. Fluorosis causes hypomineralization of the enamel which starts at the subsurface level but can extend deeper into the dentinal–enamel junction in severe cases. The development of fluorosis is very dependent on the timing, dose, and duration of fluoride exposure. The risk is lowest when the exposure happens when enamel formation has been completed. The risk increases when the exposure happens at the secretory stage, and there is even a higher risk of developing fluorosis when exposure occurs in both secretory and maturation stages (Denbesten, 1999).

8.3.2.2 Sodium lauryl sulfate

SLS is the most commonly used anionic detergent which is incorporated into toothpastes to improve their cleansing action.

It has been shown that SLS can dehydrate, cause irritation and oral mucosal desquamation, and increase the frequency of mouth ulcers in some patients (Herlofson and Barkvoll, 1996a,b). The suggested mechanism is that SLS denatures the mucin layer of the oral mucosa and exposes the underlying epithelium and therefore induces an increased risk of developing recurrent aphthous ulcers (Herlofson and Barkvoll,

1994). Therefore, it is advised to avoid using SLS-containing oral care products in patients suffering from dry mouth or sensitive mucosa.

It has also been suggested that SLS can potentially cause hypersensitivity to metal ions by increasing the mucosal permeability to sensitizing compounds. SLS has been shown in vitro to interact with the adsorption of fluoride on the enamel and therefore has the potential to reduce the efficacy of fluorides in preventing dental caries (Barkvoll, 1989). Several SLS-free toothpaste formulations have been introduced to the market to avoid the potential side effects of SLS-containing toothpastes.

8.3.2.3 Triclosan

Triclosan (2,4,4-trichloro-2-hydroxydiphenyl ether) is a broad-spectrum antibacterial agent that is incorporated into toothpastes and mouthwashes to enhance their ability to reduce plaque and improve inflammatory gingival diseases and periodontal conditions.

There have been several concerns regarding potential oral side effects of triclosan used in oral care products. In vitro experiments using monolayer cell culture systems have indicated that triclosan can induce apoptosis in human gingival fibroblasts (Zuckerbraun et al., 1998). Conversely, human and animal studies have shown that triclosan can reduce the irritation potential of SLS on oral mucosa (Baert and Veys, 1997; Skaare et al., 1997). Although allergic reactions such as contact urticaria to triclosan have been reported (Ozkaya and Kavlak Bozkurt, 2013), this material is believed to have low allergenic potential (Lachapelle, 2014).

It has been shown that triclosan can combine with chlorine in tap water to form chlorinated organics and chloroform, a known human carcinogen (Rule et al., 2005).

Concerns have been raised regarding the effects of long-term use of triclosan-containing toothpastes on the function of thyroid gland. However a recent randomized, placebo controlled clinical trial showed that triclosan toothpaste used over 4 years had no significant effect on thyroid function and suggested that 0.3% triclosan in toothpaste can be considered safe and free of significant adverse effects on the thyroid (Cullinan et al., 2012).

A recent Cochrane review which assessed the effects of triclosan-containing toothpastes in long-term control of plaque, gingivitis, and caries in children and adults concluded that there did not appear to be any serious safety concerns associated with the use of triclosan-/copolymer-containing toothpastes in studies of up to 3 years in length.

8.4 Biocompatibility of mouthwashes

8.4.1 Types of mouthwashes

Different types of mouthwashes have been developed for specific intended applications based on their main active ingredients.

Fluoride mouthwashes containing 0.05% sodium fluoride are recommended for daily use as protection against dental caries in patients with increased caries risk who require additional fluoride.

Antiplaque mouthwashes contain active antiseptic agents such as chlorhexidine, essential oils, cetylpyridinium chloride (CPC), and triclosan. Due to the side effects associated with their long-term use, antiseptic mouthwashes are recommended for short-term use in specific conditions to reduce the amount of plaque and associated inflammation.

Desensitizing mouthwashes have been developed for application by patients suffering from dentine hypersensitivity. They contain active ingredients such as potassium nitrate 3–5% or 0.8% arginine.

Biological aspects of the main active components of different types of mouthwashes are discussed below.

8.4.1.1 Chlorhexidine

Chlorhexidine is a cationic antiseptic with a bisbiguanide base and a broad-spectrum antimicrobial activity which is used in three forms: digluconate, hydrochloride, and acetate. Chlorhexidine is available as mouthrinse (0.2%), gel (1%), spray (0.2%), toothpaste (1%), root canal irrigant (2%), varnishes, and periodontal chips used as a local antimicrobial agent. Chlorhexidine mouthwash is recommended for short-term use in various clinical situations including:

- As adjunct aid to oral hygiene following periodontal treatment.
- For patients with jaw fixation following trauma or orthognathic surgery.
- In medically compromised patients: blood disorders, following chemotherapy, radiotherapy, and bone marrow transplants.
- In orthodontic appliance wearers for the first 4–8 weeks.
- For treatment of oral malodour (halitosis).

Numerous in vitro and clinical studies have investigated the efficacy of chlorhexidine in reducing plaque levels and plaque-induced gingival inflammation (Varoni et al., 2012). Cationic chlorhexidine absorbs onto the surface enamel of the tooth by binding to anionic components such as free carboxyl, sulphate, and phosphate groups as well as salivary glycoproteins. This action reduces the adhesion of proteins onto the tooth surface and therefore delays the formation of dental pellicle. Chlorhexidine also affects the colonization rate of oral bacteria on the enamel surface by coating the surface of the bacteria which results in prolonged and persistent antimicrobial action. It has been shown that a daily rinse of 10mL of 0.2% chlorhexidine mouthwash can be successful in plaque control and inhibits development of gingivitis (Loe and Schiott, 1970).

The most common oral side effects of chlorhexidine include: brown staining of teeth, mucosa, and restorations (Watts and Addy, 2001), taste disturbance (Helms et al., 1995), oral mucosal erosion, parotid swelling, and enhanced supragingival calculus formation (Varoni et al., 2012).

Rare type-I allergic reactions have been reported following oral use of chlorhexidine mouthwash. The first case was associated with the use of 1% chlorhexidine gluconate antiseptic dental gel (Thune, 1998) and the second case occurred following the use of chlorhexidine gluconate mouthwash which resulted in development of urticarial skin reaction (Sharma and Chopra, 2009). The UK Medicines and Healthcare products Regulatory Agency (MHRA) released a drug safety update in 2012 to all healthcare workers to remind them of the risk of hypersensitivity reactions associated with chlorhexidine.

Chlorhexidine gluconate has been categorized as a class B substance in terms of teratogenic potential during pregnancy due to the lack of well-controlled human studies in pregnant women. Therefore, chlorhexidine's use during pregnancy should have clear clinical justification.

8.4.1.2 Essential oils

Mouthwashes containing essential oils have been used for many years and the evidence based on several systematic reviews suggest that essential oils have almost similar short-term and long-term efficacy to chlorhexidine in reducing plaque and gingival inflammation (Gunsolley, 2010).

Commonly used essential oils in mouthwashes are thymol (0.064%), menthol (0.042%), eucalyptol (0.092%), and methyl salicylate (0.06%). Tea-tree (*Melaleuca Alternifolia*) leaf oil has also been used in some natural mouthwashes.

The most common adverse effect of essential oil mouthwashes is the complaint of altered taste. Rare allergic reactions to essential oils and reversible local reactions such as palatal erythema have also been reported (Gagari and Kabani, 1995).

Most of the clinical studies on essential oil mouthwashes have investigated the efficacy of the mouthwashes in terms of prevention of plaque and gingivitis. A recent meta-analysis of clinical trials has demonstrated clinically significant, site-specific benefits of adjunctive essential oil treatment in people within a 6-month period (Araujo et al., 2015). A comprehensive review of the literature by Vlachojannis on effectiveness and safety of essential-oil-containing mouthwashes indicated that most clinical studies have found no adverse reactions or clinical pathological changes in the oral mucosa. However, epithelial sloughing and erythema has been reported in some cases, mainly in patients suffering from dry mouth (Vlachojannis et al., 2013).

In a recent double-blind, prospective, randomized clinical trial of 80 patients (Ros-Llor and Lopez-Jornet, 2014), genotoxic effects of three different types of mouthwashes were investigated including essential oil, chlorhexidine, and triclosan-based mouthwashes. Cytogenetic analysis of the oral mucosal cells did not show any genotoxic changes or nuclear abnormalities following 2-week exposure to the mouthwashes tested in this study.

The author's research group used a three-dimensional, tissue-engineered. human oral mucosal model to assess biological effects of different types of essential oil mouthwashes. The mouthwashes tested in this study did not cause any significant mucosal toxicity as assessed by tissue viability assays, histological and ultrastructural analysis of the oral mucosa, compared with the positive control group (Moharamzadeh et al., 2009).

8.4.1.3 Alcohol

Concerns have been raised regarding the carcinogenic potential of alcohol-containing antiseptic mouthwashes. Several systematic reviews and meta-analyses have demonstrated that there is no association between ethanol-containing mouthwashes and the risk of oral cancer (McCullough and Farah, 2008; Boyle et al., 2014; Gandini et al., 2012) but a few studies have shown there is an increased risk (La Vecchia, 2009). The American Dental Association issued a statement in March 2009 saying:

> *Alcohol-containing mouthrinses are considered safe and effective in helping to prevent and reduce gingivitis and plaque when used as directed. Some individuals may be at greater risk for developing oral cancer due to life style and/or genetic factors. For this reason, it may be prudent to advise individuals that smoke, have an intolerance for alcohol (e.g. aldehyde dehydrogenase deficiency), have risk factors for developing oral cancer or a history of oral cancer to limit their use of alcohol-containing products.*

8.4.1.4 Benzydamine

Benzydamine hydrochloride is the active antiinflammatory ingredient in some mouthwashes which is used to reduce discomfort and inflammation associated with several painful conditions in the mouth, including oral ulceration, stomatitis, aphthous ulcers, radiotherapy-induced mucositis, and following oral surgery.

Studies have also demonstrated that benzydamine has some antimicrobial properties as well and can have a dual effects when combined with other therapeutic agents (Turnbull, 1995).

Although in vitro studies have suggested that benzydamine can have potential genotoxic effects on some nonhuman species (Erciyas et al., 2010), potential adverse reactions to benzydamine mouthwashes in humans may include occasional oral mucosa paresthesia and photoallergic contact dermatitis of lips and chin (Canelas et al., 2010).

8.4.1.5 Povidone iodine

Povidone iodine (polyvinylpyrrolidone-iodine) or Betadine (1%) mouthwash has been used as an antibacterial agent in the treatment of acute oral mucosal infections and also in combination with periodontal treatment and oral surgery procedures to reduce the bacterial load in the oral cavity (Greenstein, 1999).

Reported adverse reactions with the use of povidone iodine mouthwashes include:

- Local mucosal irritation and sensitivity reactions.
- Rare type-I hypersensitivity allergic reaction.
- Thyroid function impairment caused by excess iodine associated with prolonged and excessive use.
- Metabolic acidosis and impaired renal function.

8.4.1.6 Cetylpyridinium chloride

CPC, used in some types of mouthwashes (0.07%), is a cationic quaternary ammonium compound with antibacterial and antiplaque properties. Systematic reviews show that CPC-containing mouthwashes are useful oral hygiene adjuncts with additional benefits in reducing plaque and gingival inflammation (Haps et al., 2008). Side effects of CPC include staining the surface of the teeth, taste alteration, and a burning sensation (Ciancio, 1992).

8.4.1.7 Sodium bicarbonate

Sodium bicarbonate ($NaHCO_3$) does not have any direct antibacterial effect but it has a cleansing action by loosening debris and dissolving mucus. It also increases the pH in the oral cavity and prevents acidophilic bacteria overgrowth. A recent randomized clinical trial has shown that 1% sodium bicarbonate mouthwash causes less irritation to the oral mucosa in a group of sensitive oncology patients compared with some other antiseptic mouthwashes such as chlorhexidine (Choi and Kim, 2012). Other advantages of sodium bicarbonate mouthwash include low cost and ready availability in the clinic and at home for daily use.

8.4.1.8 Delmopinol

Delmopinol hydrochloride is a surface-active cationic agent that is used as the active ingredient in some mouthwashes (0.2%). It has the ability to disrupt the plaque matrix, interfere with pellicle formation, and reduce bacterial adherence.

Clinical studies have shown it is effective as an adjunct measure in reducing plaque levels and gingivitis (Addy et al., 2007).

Delmopinol's side effects are similar to those of chlorhexidine, including staining teeth and transient lingual paresthesia. However, the short-term efficacy of delmopinol is significantly lower than the efficacy of chlorhexidine in reducing oral bacterial counts (Moran et al., 1992).

8.4.1.9 Hydrogen peroxide

Hydrogen peroxide is an oxidizing agent incorporated into some mouthwashes (1.5%) which are recommended for short-term use to eradicate anaerobic bacteria found in conditions such as necrotizing ulcerative gingivitis or periodontitis. It can also have mechanical cleansing action as it produces oxygen bubbles when it comes into contact with tissues and debris.

In vitro genotoxic potential of hydrogen peroxide on bacteria and cultured cells has been demonstrated when the material comes into direct contact with living organisms. However, it does not cause any in vivo genotoxicity as metabolizing enzymes have the ability to reduce or eliminate the genotoxic effects of hydrogen peroxide (Li, 1996).

Animal studies have shown that long-term exposure to hydrogen peroxide has dose-dependent tumorigenic effects on the gastrointestinal tract (Ito et al., 1981).

Although side effects such as lingual papilla enlargement associated with long-term use of hydrogen peroxide mouthwashes have been reported, the use of low-concentration hydrogen peroxide mouthwashes is considered to be relatively safe (Walsh, 2000). Issues concerning hydrogen peroxide used in higher concentrations in tooth-whitening products are discussed below.

8.5 Biocompatibility of tooth-whitening products

8.5.1 Whitening gels

The active ingredient in most dental bleaching gels is carbamide peroxide, which produces hydrogen peroxide as it reacts with water.

The EU Cosmetic Products Regulations in 2012 prohibited the use of products containing or releasing between 0.1% and 6% hydrogen peroxide in children under 18 years of age and concentrations exceeding 6% of hydrogen peroxide remained prohibited for use in adult patients. Hydrogen peroxide at 6% is equivalent to 18% carbamide peroxide.

A comprehensive critical review by Dahl and Pallesen outlined important biological aspects of tooth-whitening (Dahl and Pallesen, 2003).

Clinical studies have shown that 10% carbamide peroxide bleaching for 5 weeks can cause increased proliferation of gingival mucosal cells (Da Costa Filho et al., 2002).

Hydrogen peroxide has a weak potential to induce local carcinogenicity possibly through DNA damage caused by releasing free radicals (Adams et al., 1996).

Over 90% satisfactory results have been reported with the use of external bleaching techniques using whitening gels (Boushell et al., 2012). Tooth sensitivity is the most common side effect of external tooth-whitening reported in up to 78% of the patients. The risk of adverse reactions increase with the use of high concentrations of above 10% peroxide. It is recommended to avoid using concentrations of above 10% carbamide peroxide for external tooth bleaching.

Studies have shown that external bleaching with 10% carbamide peroxide gel can be successfully used in the long term (up to 3 months) for the treatment of severe tetracycline staining (Tsubura, 2010).

Several studies have investigated the effects of light and heat activation on the efficacy and the incidence of side effects of whitening products (He et al., 2012). It has been shown that heat and light activation increase the risk of sensitivity in patients during vital bleaching. Also light activation does not have a statistically significant effect on the whitening efficacy of bleaching products containing high concentrations of hydrogen peroxide (Mondelli et al., 2012).

8.5.2 Whitening strips

Whitening strips contain flexible polyethylene strips which deliver 6–14% hydrogen peroxide depending on the product.

Clinical studies have shown that using whitening strips containing 6% hydrogen peroxide for 2 weeks can be safe, consistent, and as effective as external whitening with bleaching gels (Gerlach et al., 2009).

A recent meta-analysis comparing the efficacy and safety of over-the-counter whitening strips with 10% carbamide peroxide gel tray whitening has demonstrated that tooth sensitivity and gingival sensitivity were similar, regardless of the whitening method used. The observed gingival irritation was higher when the 10% carbamide peroxide gel was applied on the tray (Serraglio et al., 2016).

8.6 Biocompatibility of denture care products

8.6.1 Denture adhesives

Denture adhesives have been developed for application on the fitting surface of the dentures to improve their retention and stability. They are classified into soluble adhesives including gels, creams, powders, and nonsoluble adhesives such as pads and wafers. The most commonly used active ingredients in these products are polyvinyl methyl ether maleate copolymer (PVM-MA) and carboxymethylcellulose (CMC). Zinc and calcium salts are also added to some products to improve their adhesion.

A recent systematic review of 21 clinical studies of the efficacy of dental adhesives showed that they are effective in enhancing the retention, stability, and masticatory function of removable dentures and that they significantly improve patient satisfaction (Papadiochou et al., 2015).

Several concerns have been raised regarding the potential adverse effects of denture adhesives, but there is limited and contradictory evidence in the literature to substantiate some of these concerns as listed below:

- Microbial and fungal contamination of the adhesive: some in vitro studies have shown evidence of bacterial and fungal contamination of different denture adhesives (Gates et al., 1994) but two in vivo clinical studies have shown that there was no statistically significant difference in the population of fungal and bacterial species in oral samples taken from patients before and after the use of denture adhesives for up to 2 months (Ozkan et al., 2012; Leite et al., 2014).
- Cytotoxicity and mucosal irritation: different degrees of cytotoxicity in a dose-dependent and time-dependent manner have been associated with denture adhesives in in vitro studies using monolayer cell-culture systems (Lee et al., 2015; De Gomes et al., 2011). However, clinical and histological evaluation of oral mucosa in patients using denture adhesives have shown no inflammatory reactions or any sign of mucosal irritation in patients with good oral hygiene. Reduced thickness of the keratinized layer of the palatal mucosa has been observed with long-term use of denture adhesives (Abdelmalek and Michael, 1978). It has also been demonstrated that denture adhesive used for 6 months in patients with existing tissue irritation resulted in improvement or resolution of the symptoms (Tarbet and Grossman, 1980).
- Neurological problems associated with hypocupremia and hyperzincemia have been linked to long-term use of zinc-containing denture adhesives (Nations et al., 2008). A clinical study investigating the source of excessive zinc exposure in 11 patients suffering from copper deficiency syndrome found that these patients had been applying large amounts of zinc-containing adhesives to their ill-fitting dentures which had significantly increased their serum zinc levels and consequently decreased their serum copper levels. Following stopping the use of zinc-containing denture adhesives, these patients' copper and zinc levels returned to normal (Hedera et al., 2009).

8.7 Conclusions

Although numerous studies have investigated the efficacy and clinical performance of oral care products, there is limited high-quality evidence in terms of their biocompatibility and safety profiles. Adverse reactions to oral care products have been reported and based on the available biological data, manufacturers are constantly updating their products to enhance the efficacy and minimize their potential side effects. Clinicians should familiarize themselves with the various products available on the market, their indications for use, advantages, and potential side effects. Patients must be instructed clearly and carefully by the clinicians on the type of the product, method of use, frequency, and the duration of application of the products in each clinical situation. It is important to be aware of different susceptible groups of patients who are at greater risk of developing adverse reactions to particular oral care products and appropriate precautions to be considered when prescribing these products for the high-risk group of patients, including young children, patients with suspected allergies, pregnant patients, patients suffering from xerostomia, oncology patients receiving radiotherapy or chemotherapy, and other groups of patients discussed earlier in this chapter.

Dental care professionals are also encouraged to report any suspected adverse reactions to any of the oral care products used by their patients to help to identify potential harmful products at an early stage of postmarket surveillance.

There is a need for further research to produce high-quality evidence on the biocompatibility of currently available oral care products and to further optimize the products' formulations to reduce their potential local and systemic adverse effects while maintaining and enhancing their clinical efficacy.

References

Science brief on alcohol-containing mouthrinses and oral cancer. American Dental Association, March 2009.

Abdelmalek, R.G., Michael, C.G., 1978. The effects of denture adhesives on the palatal mucosa under complete dentures. A clinical and histological investigation. Egypt Dent. J. 24, 419–430.

Adams, S.P., Laws, G.M., Storer, R.D., Deluca, J.G., Nichols, W.W., 1996. Detection of DNA damage induced by human carcinogens in acellular assays: potential application for determining genotoxic mechanisms. Mutat. Res. 368, 235–248.

Addy, M., Moran, J., Newcombe, R.G., 2007. Meta-analyses of studies of 0.2% delmopinol mouth rinse as an adjunct to gingival health and plaque control measures. J. Clin. Periodontol. 34, 58–65.

Araujo, M.W., Charles, C.A., Weinstein, R.B., McGuire, J.A., Parikh-Das, A.M., Du, Q., et al., 2015. Meta-analysis of the effect of an essential oil-containing mouthrinse on gingivitis and plaque. J. Am. Dent. Assoc. 146, 610–622.

Baert, J.H., Veys, R.J., 1997. Triclosan inhibits sodium lauryl sulphate-induced changes in expression of cytokeratin genes in hamster cheek pouch epithelium. J. Oral Pathol. Med. 26, 181–186.

Barkvoll, P., 1989. Should toothpastes foam? Sodium lauryl sulfate—a toothpaste detergent in focus. Nor. Tannlaegeforen Tid. 99, 82–84.
Boushell, L.W., Ritter, A.V., Garland, G.E., Tiwana, K.K., Smith, L.R., Broome, A., et al., 2012. Nightguard vital bleaching: side effects and patient satisfaction 10 to 17 years post-treatment. J. Esthet. Restor. Dent. 24, 211–219.
Boyle, P., Koechlin, A., Autier, P., 2014. Mouthwash use and the prevention of plaque, gingivitis and caries. Oral Dis. 20 (Suppl. 1), 1–68.
Canelas, M.M., Cardoso, J.C., Goncalo, M., Figueiredo, A., 2010. Photoallergic contact dermatitis from benzydamine presenting mainly as lip dermatitis. Contact Dermat. 63, 85–88.
Chioca, L.R., Raupp, I.M., Da Cunha, C., Losso, E.M., Andreatini, R., 2008. Subchronic fluoride intake induces impairment in habituation and active avoidance tasks in rats. Eur. J. Pharmacol. 579, 196–201.
Choi, A.L., Sun, G., Zhang, Y., Grandjean, P., 2012. Developmental fluoride neurotoxicity: a systematic review and meta-analysis. Environ. Health Perspect. 120, 1362–1368.
Choi, S.E., Kim, H.S., 2012. Sodium bicarbonate solution versus chlorhexidine mouthwash in oral care of acute leukemia patients undergoing induction chemotherapy: a randomized controlled trial. Asian Nurs. Res. (Korean Soc. Nurs. Sci.) 6, 60–66.
Ciancio, S.G., 1992. Agents for the management of plaque and gingivitis. J. Dent. Res. 71, 1450–1454.
Cullinan, M.P., Palmer, J.E., Carle, A.D., West, M.J., Seymour, G.J., 2012. Long term use of triclosan toothpaste and thyroid function. Sci. Total Environ. 416, 75–79.
Da Costa Filho, L.C., Da Costa, C.C., Soria, M.L., Taga, R., 2002. Effect of home bleaching and smoking on marginal gingival epithelium proliferation: a histologic study in women. J. Oral Pathol. Med. 31, 473–480.
Dahl, J.E., Pallesen, U., 2003. Tooth bleaching—a critical review of the biological aspects. Crit. Rev. Oral Biol. Med. 14, 292–304.
De Gomes, P.S., Figueiral, M.H., Fernandes, M.H., Scully, C., 2011. Cytotoxicity of denture adhesives. Clin. Oral Investig. 15, 885–893.
Denbesten, P., Li, W., 2011. Chronic fluoride toxicity: dental fluorosis. Monogr. Oral Sci. 22, 81–96.
Denbesten, P.K., 1999. Biological mechanisms of dental fluorosis relevant to the use of fluoride supplements. Comm. Dent. Oral Epidemiol. 27, 41–47.
Erciyas, A.F., Erciyas, K., Sarikaya, R., 2010. Genotoxicity of two mouthwash products in the Drosophila Wing-Spot Test. Food Chem. Toxicol. 48, 2577–2580.
Gagari, E., Kabani, S., 1995. Adverse effects of mouthwash use. A review. Oral Surg. Oral Med. Oral Pathol. Oral Radiol. Endod. 80, 432–439.
Gandini, S., Negri, E., Boffetta, P., La Vecchia, C., Boyle, P., 2012. Mouthwash and oral cancer risk quantitative meta-analysis of epidemiologic studies. Ann. Agric. Environ. Med. 19, 173–180.
Gates, W.D., Goldschmidt, M., Kramer, D., 1994. Microbial contamination in four commercially available denture adhesives. J. Prosthet. Dent. 71, 154–158.
Gerlach, R.W., Barker, M.L., Karpinia, K., Magnusson, I., 2009. Single site meta-analysis of 6% hydrogen peroxide whitening strip effectiveness and safety over 2 weeks. J. Dent. 37, 360–365.
Greenstein, G., 1999. Povidone-iodine's effects and role in the management of periodontal diseases: a review. J. Periodontol. 70, 1397–1405.
Gunsolley, J.C., 2010. Clinical efficacy of antimicrobial mouthrinses. J. Dent. 38 (Suppl. 1), S6–10.

Hanks, C.T., Wataha, J.C., Sun, Z., 1996. In vitro models of biocompatibility: a review. Dent. Mater. 12, 186–193.

Haps, S., Slot, D.E., Berchier, C.E., Van der Weijden, G.A., 2008. The effect of cetylpyridinium chloride-containing mouth rinses as adjuncts to toothbrushing on plaque and parameters of gingival inflammation: a systematic review. Int. J. Dent. Hyg. 6, 290–303.

He, L.B., Shao, M.Y., Tan, K., Xu, X., Li, J.Y., 2012. The effects of light on bleaching and tooth sensitivity during in-office vital bleaching: a systematic review and meta-analysis. J. Dent. 40, 644–653.

Hedera, P., Peltier, A., Fink, J.K., Wilcock, S., London, Z., Brewer, G.J., 2009. Myelopolyneuropathy and pancytopenia due to copper deficiency and high zinc levels of unknown origin II. The denture cream is a primary source of excessive zinc. Neurotoxicology 30, 996–999.

Helms, J.A., Della-Fera, M.A., Mott, A.E., Frank, M.E., 1995. Effects of chlorhexidine on human taste perception. Arch. Oral Biol. 40, 913–920.

Herlofson, B.B., Barkvoll, P., 1994. Sodium lauryl sulfate and recurrent aphthous ulcers. A preliminary study. Acta Odontol. Scand. 52, 257–259.

Herlofson, B.B., Barkvoll, P., 1996a. The effect of two toothpaste detergents on the frequency of recurrent aphthous ulcers. Acta Odontol. Scand. 54, 150–153.

Herlofson, B.B., Barkvoll, P., 1996b. Oral mucosal desquamation caused by two toothpaste detergents in an experimental model. Eur. J. Oral Sci. 104, 21–26.

Ito, A., Watanabe, H., Naito, M., Naito, Y., 1981. Induction of duodenal tumors in mice by oral administration of hydrogen peroxide. Gan 72, 174–175.

La Vecchia, C., 2009. Mouthwash and oral cancer risk: an update. Oral Oncol. 45, 198–200.

Lachapelle, J.M., 2014. A comparison of the irritant and allergenic properties of antiseptics. Eur. J. Dermatol. 24, 3–9.

Lee, Y., Ahn, J.S., Yi, Y.A., Chung, S.H., Yoo, Y.J., Ju, S.W., et al., 2015. Cytotoxicity of four denture adhesives on human gingival fibroblast cells. Acta Odontol. Scand. 73, 87–92.

Leite, A.R., Mendoza-Marin, D.O., Paleari, A.G., Rodriguez, L.S., Roccia, A.A., Policastro, V.B., et al., 2014. Crossover clinical trial of the influence of the use of adhesive on biofilm formation. J. Prosthet. Dent. 112, 349–356.

Li, Y., 1996. Biological properties of peroxide-containing tooth whiteners. Food Chem. Toxicol. 34, 887–904.

Loe, H., Schiott, C.R., 1970. The effect of mouthrinses and topical application of chlorhexidine on the development of dental plaque and gingivitis in man. J. Periodontal. Res. 5, 79–83.

McCullough, M.J., Farah, C.S., 2008. The role of alcohol in oral carcinogenesis with particular reference to alcohol-containing mouthwashes. Aust. Dent. J. 53, 302–305.

Moharamzadeh, K., Brook, I.M., Van Noort, R., Scutt, A.M., Thornhill, M.H., 2007. Tissue-engineered oral mucosa: a review of the scientific literature. J. Dent. Res. 86, 115–124.

Moharamzadeh, K., Brook, I.M., Scutt, A.M., Thornhill, M.H., Van Noort, R., 2008a. Mucotoxicity of dental composite resins on a tissue-engineered human oral mucosal model. J. Dent. 36, 331–336.

Moharamzadeh, K., Brook, I.M., Van Noort, R., Scutt, A.M., Smith, K.G., Thornhill, M.H., 2008b. Development, optimization and characterization of a full-thickness tissue engineered human oral mucosal model for biological assessment of dental biomaterials. J. Mater. Sci. Mater. Med. 19, 1793–1801.

Moharamzadeh, K., Franklin, K.L., Brook, I.M., Van Noort, R., 2009. Biologic assessment of antiseptic mouthwashes using a three-dimensional human oral mucosal model. J. Periodontol. 80, 769–775.

Moharamzadeh, K., Colley, H., Murdoch, C., Hearnden, V., Chai, W.L., Brook, I.M., et al., 2012. Tissue-engineered oral mucosa. J. Dent. Res. 91, 642–650.
Mondelli, R.F., Azevedo, J.F., Francisconi, A.C., Almeida, C.M., Ishikiriama, S.K., 2012. Comparative clinical study of the effectiveness of different dental bleaching methods – two year follow-up. J. Appl. Oral Sci. 20, 435–443.
Moran, J., Addy, M., Wade, W.G., Maynard, J.H., Roberts, S.E., Astrom, M., et al., 1992. A comparison of delmopinol and chlorhexidine on plaque regrowth over a 4-day period and salivary bacterial counts. J. Clin. Periodontol. 19, 749–753.
Nations, S.P., Boyer, P.J., Love, L.A., Burritt, M.F., Butz, J.A., Wolfe, G.I., et al., 2008. Denture cream: an unusual source of excess zinc, leading to hypocupremia and neurologic disease. Neurology 71, 639–643.
Ozkan, Y.K., Ucankale, M., Ozcan, M., Uner, N., 2012. Effect of denture adhesive on the micro-organisms in vivo. Gerodontology 29, 9–16.
Ozkaya, E., Kavlak Bozkurt, P., 2013. An unusual case of triclosan-induced immunological contact urticaria. Contact Dermat. 68, 121–123.
Papadiochou, S., Emmanouil, I., Papadiochos, I., 2015. Denture adhesives: a systematic review. J. Prosthet. Dent. 113, 391–397. e2.
Ros-Llor, I., Lopez-Jornet, P., 2014. Cytogenetic analysis of oral mucosa cells, induced by chlorhexidine, essential oils in ethanolic solution and triclosan mouthwashes. Environ. Res. 132, 140–145.
Rule, K.L., Ebbett, V.R., Vikesland, P.J., 2005. Formation of chloroform and chlorinated organics by free-chlorine-mediated oxidation of triclosan. Environ. Sci. Technol. 39, 3176–3185.
Serraglio, C.R., Zanella, L., Dalla-Vecchia, K.B., Rodrigues-Junior, S.A., 2016. Efficacy and safety of over-the-counter whitening strips as compared to home-whitening with 10% carbamide peroxide gel-systematic review of RCTs and metanalysis. Clin. Oral Investig. 20, 1–14.
Sharma, A., Chopra, H., 2009. Chlorhexidine urticaria: a rare occurrence with a common mouthwash. Indian J. Dent. Res. 20, 377–379.
Shulman, J.D., Wells, L.M., 1997. Acute fluoride toxicity from ingesting home-use dental products in children, birth to 6 years of age. J. Public Health Dent. 57, 150–158.
Skaare, A.B., Rolla, G., Barkvoll, P., 1997. The influence of triclosan, zinc or propylene glycol on oral mucosa exposed to sodium lauryl sulphate. Eur. J. Oral Sci. 105, 527–533.
Tarbet, W.J., Grossman, E., 1980. Observations of denture-supporting tissue during six months of denture adhesive wearing. J. Am. Dent. Assoc. 101, 789–791.
Thune, P., 1998. Two patients with chlorhexidine allergy–anaphylactic reactions and eczema. Tidsskr Nor Laegeforen 118, 3295–3296.
Tsubura, S., 2010. Clinical evaluation of three months' nightguard vital bleaching on tetracycline-stained teeth using Polanight 10% carbamide gel: 2-year follow-up study. Odontology 98, 134–138.
Turnbull, R.S., 1995. Benzydamine Hydrochloride (Tantum) in the management of oral inflammatory conditions. J. Can. Dent. Assoc. 61, 127–134.
Varoni, E., Tarce, M., Lodi, G., Carrassi, A., 2012. Chlorhexidine (CHX) in dentistry: state of the art. Minerva. Stomatol. 61, 399–419.
Vlachojannis, C., Winsauer, H., Chrubasik, S., 2013. Effectiveness and safety of a mouthwash containing essential oil ingredients. Phytother. Res. 27, 685–691.
Walsh, L.J., 2000. Safety issues relating to the use of hydrogen peroxide in dentistry. Aust. Dent. J. 45, 257–269. quiz 289.

Watts, A., Addy, M., 2001. Tooth discolouration and staining: a review of the literature. Br. Dent. J. 190, 309–316.
Whitford, G.M., 1987. Fluoride in dental products: safety considerations. J. Dent. Res. 66, 1056–1060.
Whitford, G.M., 2011. Acute toxicity of ingested fluoride. Monogr. Oral Sci. 22, 66–80.
Williams, D.F., 1987. Definitions in Biomaterials. Elsevier, Oxford.
Zuckerbraun, H.L., Babich, H., May, R., Sinensky, M.C., 1998. Triclosan: cytotoxicity, mode of action, and induction of apoptosis in human gingival cells in vitro. Eur. J. Oral Sci. 106, 628–636.

Index

Note: Page numbers followed by "*f*" and "*t*" refer to figures and tables, respectively.

FSC
www.fsc.org
MIX
Papier | Fördert
gute Waldnutzung
FSC® C083411

Kolibri 360 GmbH
Ferdinand-Jühlke-Straße 7
99095 Erfurt, Deutschland
produktsicherheit@kolibri360.de